VETERINARY
Instruments and Equipment

T0308347

VETERINARY
Instruments and Equipment
A POCKET GUIDE

Fifth Edition

Teresa F. Sonsthagen, BS, LVT
Senior Lecturer, Co-Director of the Veterinary Technology Program, Retired
North Dakota State University
Fargo, North Dakota

ELSEVIER

Elsevier
3251 Riverport Lane
St. Louis, Missouri 63043

Veterinary Instruments and Equipment: A Pocket Guide, Fifth edition.   ISBN 978-0-443-11707-7

Copyright © 2025 by Elsevier Inc. All rights are reserved, including those for text and data mining, AI training, and similar technologies.

Publisher's note: Elsevier takes a neutral position with respect to territorial disputes or jurisdictional claims in its published content, including in maps and institutional affiliations.

No part of this publication may be reproduced or transmitted in any form or by any means, electronic or mechanical, including photocopying, recording, or any information storage and retrieval system, without permission in writing from the publisher. Details on how to seek permission, further information about the Publisher's permissions policies and our arrangements with organizations such as the Copyright Clearance Center and the Copyright Licensing Agency, can be found at our website: www.elsevier.com/permissions.

This book and the individual contributions contained in it are protected under copyright by the Publisher (other than as may be noted herein).

Notice

Practitioners and researchers must always rely on their own experience and knowledge in evaluating and using any information, methods, compounds or experiments described herein. Because of rapid advances in the medical sciences, in particular, independent verification of diagnoses and drug dosages should be made. To the fullest extent of the law, no responsibility is assumed by Elsevier, authors, editors or contributors for any injury and/or damage to persons or property as a matter of products liability, negligence or otherwise, or from any use or operation of any methods, products, instructions, or ideas contained in the material herein.

Content Strategist: Melissa Rawe, Samantha Hart
Senior Content Development Specialist: Vaishali Singh
Publishing Services Manager: Deepthi Unni
Senior Project Manager: Manchu Mohan
Senior Book Designer: Brian Salisbury

Printed in India

Last digit is the print number: 9 8 7 6 5 4 3 2 1

Working together
to grow libraries in
developing countries

www.elsevier.com • www.bookaid.org

Preface

Becoming familiar with veterinary instruments and equipment is a vital part of the veterinary technology curriculum. To become a valuable member of the clinical team, it is crucial that students learn to recognize individual veterinary instruments, their main function, and their special characteristics.

This book was developed to help students who may not have access to these instruments when they are ready to study. A firm grasp of how these instruments are used increases the useful life span of the instruments and prevents injuries from improper use.

This book was designed in a flash card format so that one can flip the book to separate the picture from the name and descriptions. This allows students to quiz themselves. This self-study tool features instruments and equipment used in all aspects of veterinary medicine.

The book is organized into two parts. Restraint, medical, and diagnostic instruments are covered in the first part. Surgical instruments are covered in the second part and are organized, beginning with general surgical instruments and proceeding to specialized instruments for orthopedic and ophthalmic procedures.

The original list of instruments and equipment to be included was reviewed by veterinary technician educators from all parts of the United States and Canada, and many were added at their suggestion. If any have been missed, it is not for lack of trying, but let us know if you have ideas for others to include in the next edition.

Be sure to check out the Evolve site accompanying this edition, with its updated image collection, timed instrument quizzes, and the image library, with selected instruments that you can zoom in to and rotate. Register now at http://evolve.elsevier.com/Sonsthagen/instruments/

Teresa F. Sonsthagen, BS, LVT

Acknowledgments

I would like to take this opportunity to acknowledge Hans Jorgensen, DVM, Jorgensen Laboratories, Inc.; Liz Bowie, Nasco; Mac Everett and Lora Rios, Miltex; Victor Colon and Harry Wotton, Securos; Goldway, Inc.; Mark Helbling, L & H Branding Irons; Jennifer Zdesar, Dr. Bretts Pets; Tabetha Ketzner, No-Bull Enterprises LLC; Mikel Galicia, Allflex/Merck Animal Health; Amy Paulic, Arrowquip; Woody Sherwood, Stone Manufacturing; Scott Johnson, Kane Manufacturing; Lauren, Bella Veterinary Products; Scott Lyons, EXEL International; Bill Berkelmans, Berkelmans Welding & Manufacturing Inc.; Zoetis Veterinary; Ed Szymanski, Diamond Farrier Company; John Lynch, Sydell Inc.; Julie Garella, MacKinnon Products, LLC; Joe Hecker and Scott, Diagnostic Imaging Systems; and Karen Herdon, Midmark. They all contributed wonderful pictures for this book, ensuring its completeness.

Contents

PART 1

General Medical Instruments and Restraint Equipment

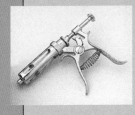

CHAPTER 1

Instruments for the Administration of Medicine and Sampling

This chapter describes the instruments that are used to deliver medications or draw blood, urine, and tissue samples from the body.

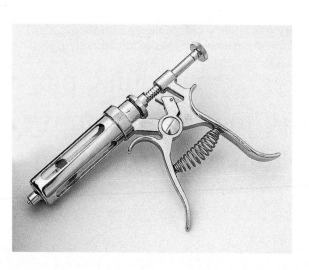

INSTRUMENT Automatic Dose Syringe

Large animal species

FUNCTION To administer intramuscular (IM) or subcutaneous (SQ) injections to multiple animals without reloading the syringe.

COMMON NAME Automatic syringe

CHARACTERISTICS A syringe barrel is attached to a handle with a dial that can be set to deliver 1 to 5 mL at a time with a squeeze of the handle. Care must be taken to clean the syringe thoroughly to prevent drug interactions and the spread of disease. The rubber gaskets inside the syringe must be oiled with mineral oil to keep them pliable.

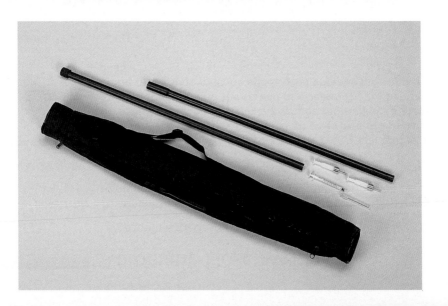

Blow Dart Syringe

All species

FUNCTION To propel a dart syringe toward an animal that is too wild or ferocious to handle.

CHARACTERISTICS This hollow tube is designed to accommodate a special syringe that flies by air propulsion and discharges on impact. The tube usually has a mouthpiece on one end. It is often used to administer an anesthetic to animals from a safe distance.

8

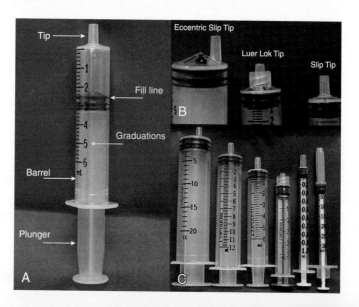

Disposable Syringes

All species

FUNCTION To administer parenteral medications or to draw blood or other fluids from the body.

COMMON NAME Syringe

CHARACTERISTICS Plastic syringes are made of three parts. (A). The tip is the part to which a needle can be attached, and it can fit into the hub of a catheter. The tip is available in three types (B). A slip tip can be centered, or it can be eccentric, meaning it is positioned to one side of the barrel; a Luer-Lok tip has threads onto which a needle hub can be turned and locked into place. The barrel determines the size and is marked with graduations to measure

Disposable Syringes (continued)

the solutions to be delivered. The plunger has a rubber stopper on the end of a shaft, which pulls or pushes the solutions into or out of the syringe. The rubber stopper, as indicated, is also used as a fill guide by lining it up with the graduations. Image C shows samples of different sizes of syringes and their corresponding graduations.

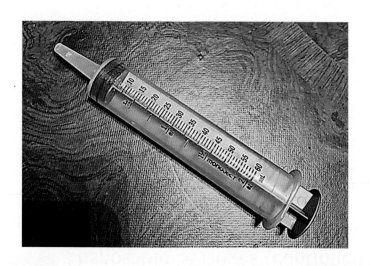

Disposable Syringes—Catheter-Style Tip

All species

FUNCTION To administer liquid medication or food through the tip of a feeding tube. Can also be used to rinse the oral cavity free of debris or flush a wound cavity.

COMMON NAME Catheter-tip syringe

CHARACTERISTICS Usually, a 60-mL syringe with a long tapered tip that can be placed at the end of a urinary catheter or feeding tube. It can also be used to rinse the mouth or wound cavity free of debris.

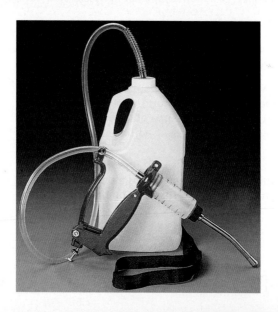

Dose Syringe—Drench-Matic

Large animal species

FUNCTION To administer oral liquid medications without multiple reloading of the syringe.

CHARACTERISTICS The syringe has a hose that goes to a tankard; with each squeeze of the handle, the exact amount of medication is delivered orally. Note the oral nozzle attached to the barrel, which can be exchanged for different sizes per animal species.

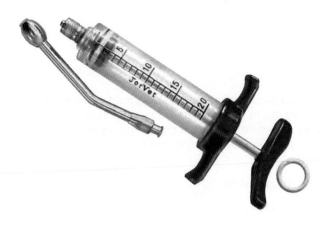

Dose Syringe—Nylon Syringe Sheep and Goat

Large animal species

FUNCTION To administer liquid medication orally.

COMMON NAME Drenching syringe, drencher

CHARACTERISTICS Made of durable nylon, this syringe is easy to take apart, clean, and sterilize. The Luer-Lok fitting accepts the oral drench nozzles, and the barrel will hold 150 cc. To fill, depress the plunger, insert the nozzle into liquid, and then pull back on the plunger.

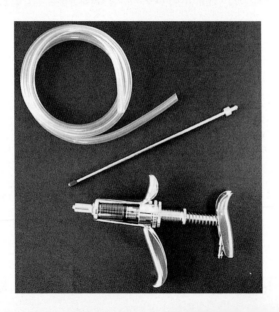

Dose Syringe—Vetamatic Large Animal Species

FUNCTION To administer IM or SQ injections to multiple animals with automatic reloading of the syringe.

CHARACTERISTICS This syringe has an attachment for a hose that is connected to a tankard or to a collapsible bottle. When the plunger is pushed in, the medication or vaccine is delivered; when it is released, it draws in the preselected amount from the tankard or bottle.

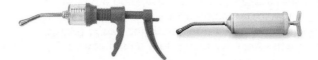

Dosing/Rinsing Syringes

Large animal species

FUNCTION To administer liquid medications orally or to rinse the oral cavity of debris.

COMMON NAME Drenching syringe, drencher or rinsing syringe

CHARACTERISTICS Both syringes can be filled with medication, water, or other solutions to be used as a rinsing agent to clean the oral cavity or as a drenching gun. The pistol grip syringe can be purchased in various sizes. The dose is adjusted by turning the bottom handle, and the Labelvage syringe can be adjusted to 50-mL increments. Both dispense the fluid by pushing down the plunger.

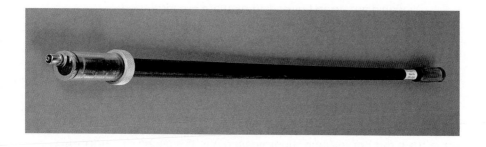

Pole Syringe

All species

FUNCTION To administer a parenteral injection to an animal too wild or ferocious to handle.

CHARACTERISTICS The plunger of a syringe is attached to a long pole. A regular syringe is taken apart, and the barrel is attached to the plunger of the pole syringe. The syringe is filled in the normal way, and the handler uses the pole to insert the needle and push the plunger from a safe distance. The plunger section can be changed to accommodate various syringe sizes. These are often used to administer an anesthetic.

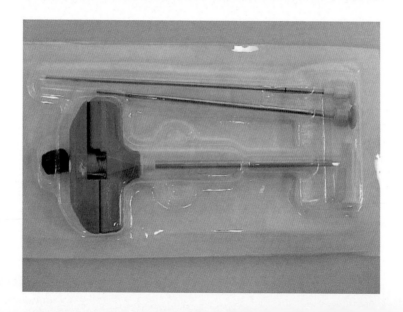

INSTRUMENT # Biopsy Needle—Bone Marrow

Small animal species

FUNCTION To perform biopsies of the marrow, not the bone.

CHARACTERISTICS This needle has a large handle that facilitates the introduction of the needle through the bone. It also has a stylet to prevent tissue coring.

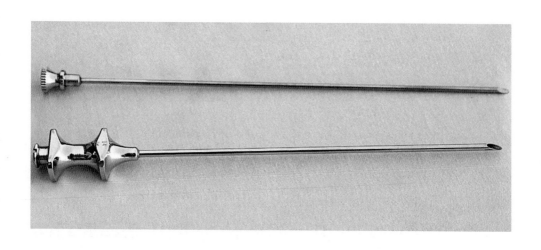

Biopsy Needle—Modified Silverman

Small animal species

FUNCTION To perform biopsies.

CHARACTERISTICS A small handle facilitates the introduction of the needle; a stylet prevents premature coring.

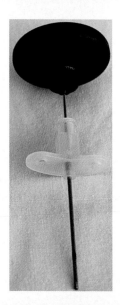

Bone Marrow Intraosseous Needle

Small and exotic animal species

FUNCTION To perform intraosseous infusion in small animals or birds. It can be used on animals that are hypovolemic, which makes finding a vein difficult.

CHARACTERISTICS An over-the-needle cannula can be left in place once the needle is withdrawn. The most common spot for the introduction of this needle is the proximal femur.

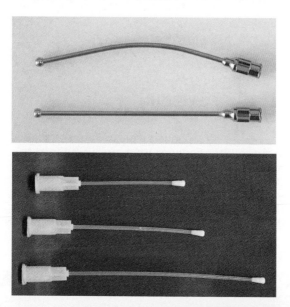

Feeding and Dosing Needles

Small and exotic animal species

FUNCTION To stomach-feed small animals, such as rodents, birds, and reptiles.

COMMON NAME Gavage needle, dosing needle, flushing needle

CHARACTERISTICS The needles have blunted, round tips that can be inserted into the esophagus to deliver nutrients, washes, or medications directly to the stomach. They are usually 2 to 3 inches long and are either straight or curved. There are new flexible dosing needles that have multiple uses.

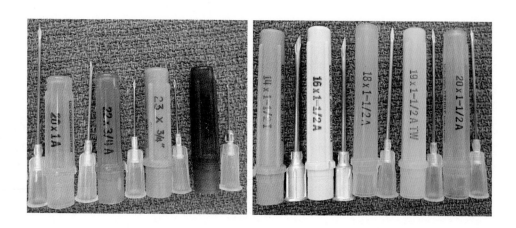

INSTRUMENT Hypodermic Needles

All species

FUNCTION To inject parenteral medications.

COMMON NAME Needles

CHARACTERISTICS Stainless steel shafts have plastic or aluminum hubs. They come in various lengths and gauges. The following is a list of gauges, from the smallest lumen size to the largest, and their general uses. Different brands have different-colored covers; it is advisable to learn these colors so that in an emergency situation, identification can be quick.

Hypodermic Needles (continued)

25- TO 30-GAUGE NEEDLES

Needles of these sizes are usually used on very small animals: birds, reptiles, pocket pets, kittens, and puppies. They can also be used for intradermal injections, tuberculosis and allergy testing, and the delivery of local anesthetics. The lengths of these needles are usually less than 1 inch and range from 1/2 inch to 5/8 inch.

23- AND 22-GAUGE NEEDLES

Needles of these sizes are usually used for general injections in dogs and cats. The 22-gauge needle is the standard size found in most clinics and is used for injections and drawing blood. The lengths of these needles usually range from 5/8 inch to 1 inch, but 1½-inch needles can also be found.

Hypodermic Needles (continued)

20-, 19-, AND 18-GAUGE NEEDLES

Needles of these sizes are usually used in large dogs such as Great Danes and Saint Bernards and in sheep, goats, cattle, and horses. Those used in larger animals may be as long as 1½ inches, as opposed to the standard 1 inch.

16- AND 14-GAUGE NEEDLES

These two needles are not used frequently; however, they can be found in most large or mixed animal clinics. They are useful for delivering large volumes of intravenous fluids quickly. They are also useful when a very thick substance must be injected and the patient is uncooperative.

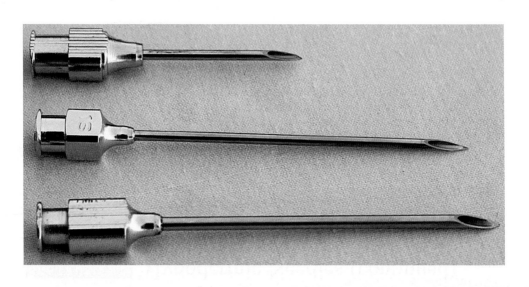

Hypodermic Needle—Stainless Steel

FUNCTION To deliver parenteral medications.

COMMON NAME Needle, nondisposable needle, stainless steel needle, bleeding needle

CHARACTERISTICS Stainless steel needles come in various lengths and gauges. The most common sizes are 14-, 16-, and 18-gauge needles at 1½ inches to 3 inches in length. The advantage of these needles is that they can be used again after sterilization. The disadvantages are that they lose their sharp edge and must be sharpened manually, and if improperly sterilized, they may spread diseases such as malignant catarrhal fever, warts, and leukosis.

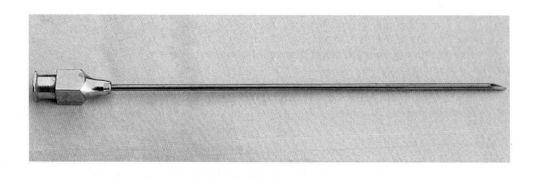

Hypodermic Needle—Swine-Bleeding Needle—4-Inch, 18-Gauge

Large animal species

FUNCTION To draw blood from the anterior vena cava of a pig.

CHARACTERISTICS A 4-inch stainless steel needle with a standard hub. The needle must be cleaned or at least rinsed soon after use because blood clots inside the needle lumen make it unusable.

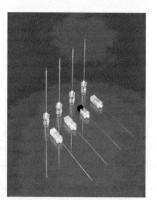

Disposable Spinal Needles

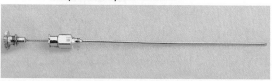

Stainless Steel Spinal Needle

Spinal Needles—Disposable and Stainless Steel

All species

FUNCTION To perform aspiration biopsies and drainage procedures.

CHARACTERISTICS This needle has a shorter bevel length than a standard needle; it also has a matched ground bevel that eliminates the possibility of tissue coring.

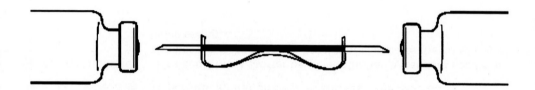

INSTRUMENT Transfer Needle

FUNCTION To transfer the liquid contents from one bottle to another without the use of a syringe.

CHARACTERISTICS The double-ended needle can aseptically pierce the rubber stoppers on the bottles.

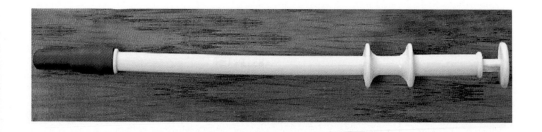

Subcategory—Small Animal

Pet piller

FUNCTION To orally deliver solid medication to small animals.

COMMON NAME Pilling gun

CHARACTERISTICS A plunger reaches through the shaft of the instrument and ends with a flared receptacle for pills. It is a small version of the balling gun.

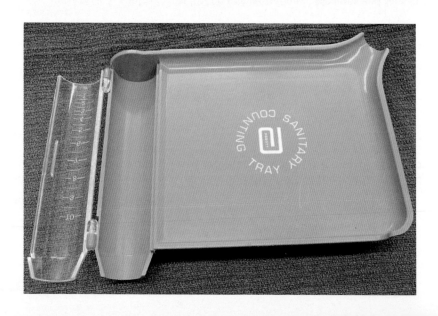

INSTRUMENT Pill-Counting Tray

FUNCTION To count out several pills without touching them with the bare hand.

CHARACTERISTICS A flat spill tray is attached to a trough with a cover. The pills are spilled onto the tray, and as they are counted out, they are pushed into the trough. Once the proper number to fill the prescription is in the trough, the cover is closed. One corner of the tray is an open funnel that allows excess pills to be put back into the bottle. The opposite corner has an opening at the cover end of the trough; this allows the counted pills to be put into a dispensing envelope or bottle to send home with the client.

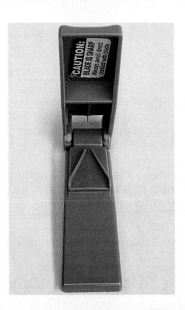

Pill Splitter

FUNCTION   To split tablets accurately for appropriate doses.

CHARACTERISTICS   A square or a round plastic holder allows one pill to be placed in a wedge-shaped groove. The lid on the holder contains a razor blade that, when the lid closes, cuts the tablet in half or in quarters.

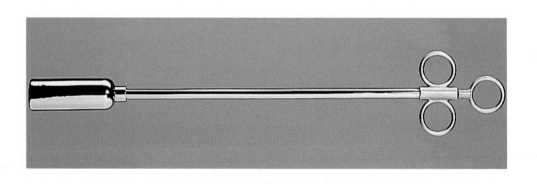

Subcategory—Large Animal

Balling gun

FUNCTION To deliver solid medication orally to large animals.

CHARACTERISTICS A plunger reaches through the shaft of the instrument and ends in a flared receptacle for a pill or bolus. Some guns have springs inside the receptacle to hold the bolus in place. The gun is pushed down the throat, and once past the esophageal groove, the plunger is pushed to send the bolus the rest of the way down the esophagus. The receptacle comes in 5⁄8-inch, 7⁄8-inch, and 1-inch diameters. Some models have interchangeable heads that screw on and off.

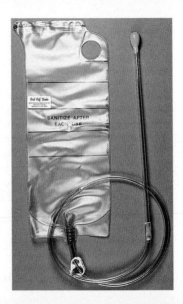

Oral Calf Drencher

FUNCTION To give large amounts of oral fluids to calves, foals, or lambs.

COMMON NAME Calf drencher, oral drencher, calf bag

CHARACTERISTICS A large reservoir bag ends in a drenching wand. The wand is passed into the esophagus, and gravity causes the bag to empty.

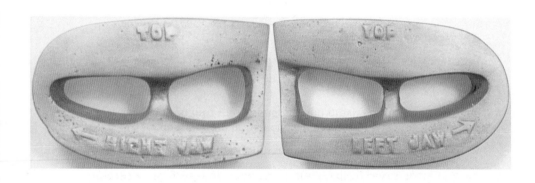

Speculum—Drinkwater

FUNCTION To hold the mouth open to pass a stomach tube.

CHARACTERISTICS A flat bar with a hole large enough to accommodate a stomach tube, balling gun, or drench syringe is placed in the mouth. This can be used in cattle, sheep, and goats; the smaller version can be used in small animals.

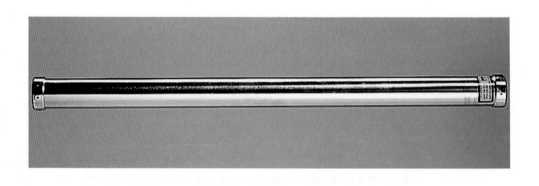

Speculum—Frick

FUNCTION Used on large animals to hold the jaws open wide enough to enable the passage of the stomach tube down the throat.

CHARACTERISTICS A stainless steel tube that is approximately 19½ inches long.

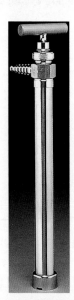

Stomach or Drench Pump

FUNCTION   To pump medication through the stomach tube into the stomach.

COMMON NAME   Stomach pump

CHARACTERISTICS   A stainless steel pump with a handle at the top performs the pumping; an adapter for the stomach tube can be attached to the pump. Once the tube is in place, it is attached to the pump. The operator pulls up the handle to load the pump and pushes it down to deliver the medication through the tube.

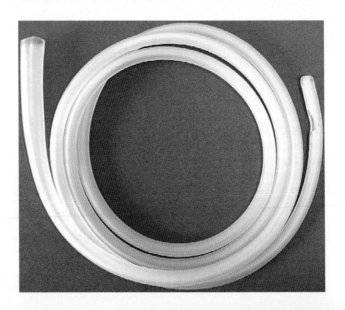

INSTRUMENT Stomach Tube

FUNCTION To deliver liquid medications directly to the stomach via the esophagus; also used to relieve gas from the rumen in cases of moderate bloat.

CHARACTERISTICS Long red rubber or polypropylene tubes come in various diameters and lengths. Inside diameters and lengths are 1/4 inch × 7 feet, 5/16 inch × 9 feet, 3/8 inch × 9 feet, and 1/2 inch × 10 feet.

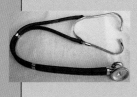

CHAPTER 2

Diagnostic Instruments

This chapter covers instruments that assist in the general
evaluation of patient health status.

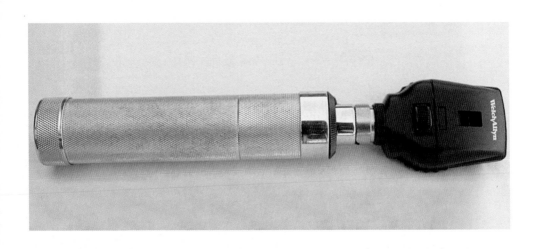

Ophthalmoscope

FUNCTION To view the external and internal structures of the eyeball.

CHARACTERISTICS The head of the ophthalmoscope has one dial that controls the amount and shape of light and another dial that controls the depth of penetration. Many handles can be used interchangeably with an otoscope head. The handles can be battery operated or plugged in to be recharged. The user turns on the light by depressing the red button and turning the black dial.

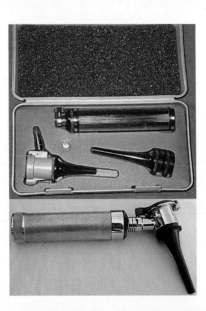

Otoscope

FUNCTION To view the internal structures of the ear canal and eardrum.

CHARACTERISTICS The head of an otoscope has a light source and cones of varying lengths and diameters that fit inside the ear canal. The cones can be changed by slipping them into the ring receptacle. To control the light, the user depresses the red button and turns the black dial. Many otoscopes have a magnifying glass to assist viewing. With the attached otoscope cones, it can also be used to illuminate the vaginal vault in female dogs and cats.

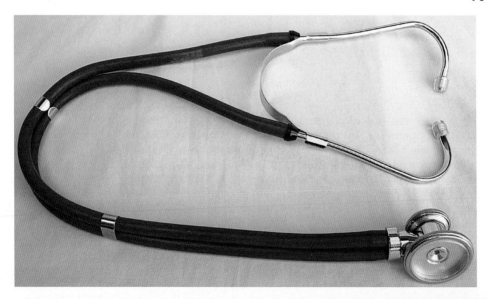

Stethoscope

FUNCTION To auscultate the heart, lungs, and digestive organs.

CHARACTERISTICS The head is equipped with a single or dual bell covered by a tight plastic membrane attached to a long rubber tube that ends in earpieces. If the head has dual bells, the user can engage one or the other by simply turning the bell in a circular motion. The bells allow for the auscultation of high- and low-frequency noises.

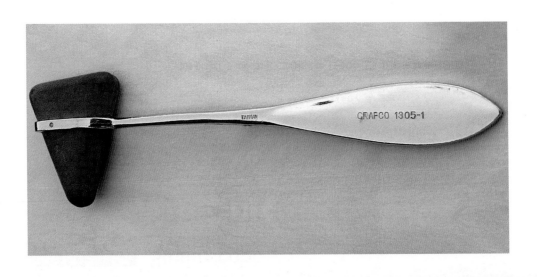

INSTRUMENT Taylor Percussion Hammer

FUNCTION To perform a neurologic examination.

CHARACTERISTICS A triangular rubber hammer is used to strike nerve points gently and judge the animal's reaction.

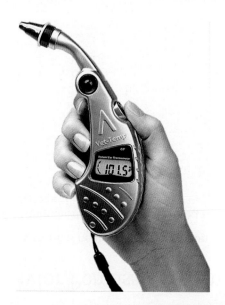

Thermometer: Aural (Vet Temp)

FUNCTION To determine the body temperature of an animal.

CHARACTERISTICS A small animal's temperature is taken by placing a short probe into the ear canal. This method is fast and seems to be accurate. The user should watch for signs that the batteries are getting low.

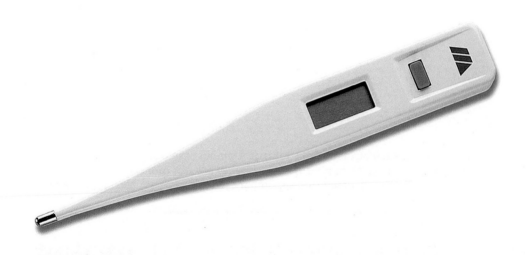

Thermometer: Digital

FUNCTION   To determine the body temperature of an animal.

CHARACTERISTICS   Housed in plastic and equipped with a small window that displays the temperature, this thermometer has a long, skinny tip that can be inserted easily into the rectum. Most of these thermometers beep when they have achieved their readings. When compared with the reading of a glass thermometer, that of a digital thermometer can vary by a degree or two, so checking it against the reading of a glass thermometer is advisable. If a wide range of readings is found in an animal assumed to be healthy, the thermometer's batteries may be low and should be replaced.

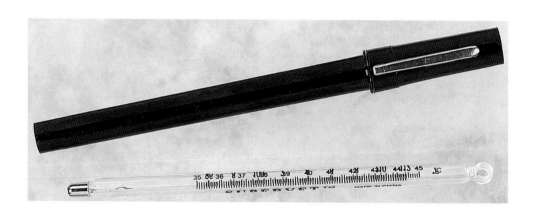

Thermometer: Mercury

Small and Large Animals

FUNCTION To determine the body temperature of an animal.

CHARACTERISTICS A glass tube is filled with mercury and has graduations from 94°F to 110°F on large-animal thermometers and 96°F to 105°F on small-animal thermometers. The small-animal thermometer is usually 4 inches long; the large-animal thermometer is 5 inches long and is topped by a ring. The ring allows the user to attach a string and a clip, which in turn are attached to the hair on the tail of a horse or cow. This prevents the thermometer from falling to the ground if the animal defecates. Both thermometers are inserted into the rectum for approximately 2 minutes to obtain an optimal reading.

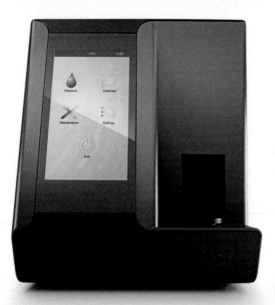

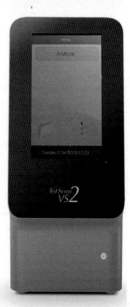

Vetscan HM5

Vetscan VS2

INSTRUMENT

Analyzers and Imagyst Scanner—Zoetis

All species

FUNCTION Vetscan HM5 is an automated hematology analyzer that provides the complete blood count. The Vetscan VS2 is a blood chemistry analyzer. When connected to the Imagyst, which is an artificial intelligence scanner, it can produce morphological data for not only blood smears, but it will also scan dermatology smears and parasitology results from a fecal slide. The Vetscan UA reads the urine strips and calculates the protein:creatinine ratio and microalbumin levels. When combined with the Vetscan Small Animal Sediment Analyzer (not shown), it will provide

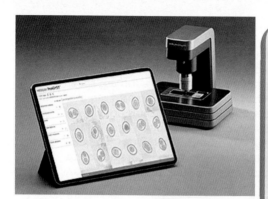

Vetscan Imagyst

Vetscan UA

Vetscan Witness

Analyzers and Imagyst Scanner— Zoetis (continued)

sedimentation results. The Vetscan Witness and Rapid Test is a rapid test for *Dirofilaria immitis*; *Anaplasma phagocytophilum* and *Anaplasma platys*; *Borrelia burgdorferi*; and *Ehrlichia canis*, *Ehrlichia chaffeensis*, and *Ehrlichia ewingii* in canines.

CHARACTERISTICS This is just one of many types of analyzers available for the veterinary market. They all provide quick and accurate laboratory results.

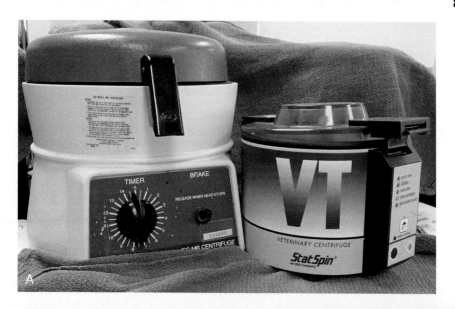

Centrifuge

FUNCTION   Equipment used to separate different components from body fluids.

CHARACTERISTICS   All centrifuges spin at various speeds creating centrifugal force, which pushes the heavier components to the bottom of the sample tube. (A) Centrifuge *(left)* used for hematocrits that use small, thin glass tubes. A StatSpin centrifuge *(right)* accomodates small tubes that are ideal for bird and rodent samples. (B) The orange SeroSpin will accommodate 3-mL vacuum tubes. (C) This is a "fixed head" centrifuge, meaning the tubes do not move. (D) This is a "slant head" centrifuge, meaning the tubes swing out with the centrifugal force. Both (C) and (D) accommodate 15-mL test tubes and have either plugs or interchangeable racks that hold 3- to 5-mL tubes as well.

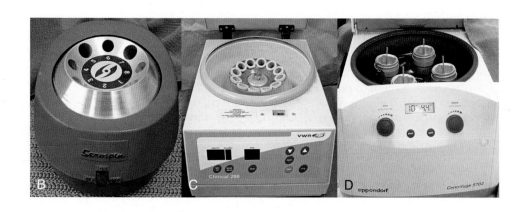

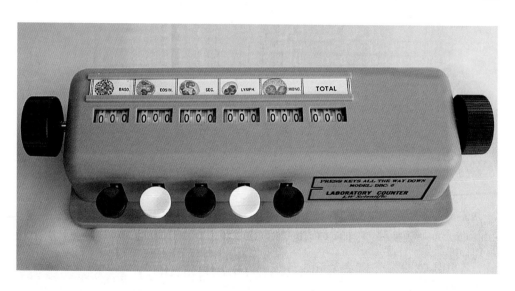

Differential Cell Counter

FUNCTION To aid in the counting of the white and red blood cells, platelets, and sperm.

COMMON NAME Cell counter

CHARACTERISTICS A five- or seven-button tally counter is labeled with the various types of blood cells seen on a differential. As the user finds each cell on the slide, the appropriate button is pushed; each push counts as one cell. A bell rings when 100 cells have been counted.

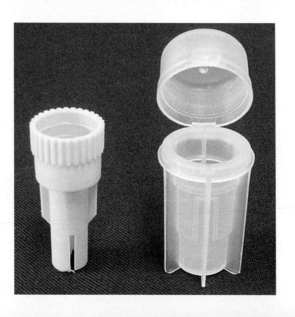

Fecalyzers

FUNCTION To set up a fecal test for the presence of parasites.

CHARACTERISTICS A small receptacle is filled with feces; a tube is placed on top and filled with fecal solution. The feces and solution are mixed thoroughly and then filled to the brim. A coverslip is placed on top of the filled tube and allowed to rest for a minimum of 10 minutes. The parasite eggs float to the top and adhere to the coverslip.

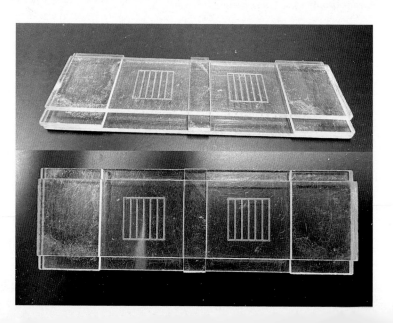

Hemocytometer

FUNCTION To aid in the counting of white and red blood cells, platelets, and sperm.

CHARACTERISTICS This glass instrument is etched with grids and has two fill apertures. A grid or a combination of grids is used to count the cells or sperm.

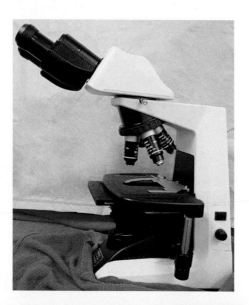

Microscope

FUNCTION An instrument used to magnify minute objects.

CHARACTERISTICS The binocular microscope shown has four objectives that magnify objects by 4×, 10×, 40×, and 100× the power of the ocular, which is usually 10×. This means that an object under 4× is magnified by $4 \times 10 = 400$ times, all the way up to $100 \times 10 = 1000$ times. The 100× is used with oil immersion to clarify the object. Bacteria, blood, and tissue cells are usually looked at under 100×.

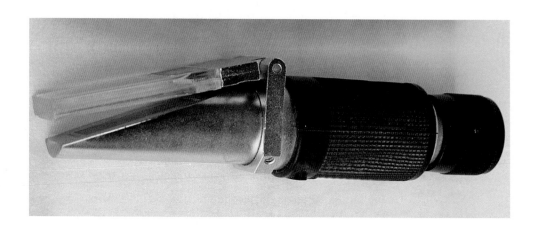

Refractometer

FUNCTION To measure total solids in plasma and specific gravity in urine.

CHARACTERISTICS An eyepiece is attached to one end and a glass pad with a plastic cover is on the other end. The user fills the glass pad and reads the scales, which can be viewed through the eyepiece.

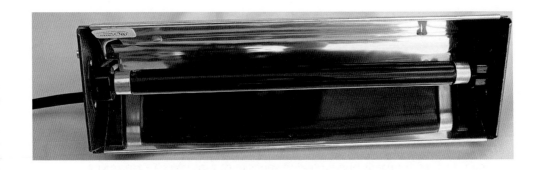

Wood Light

FUNCTION To confirm or rule out the possibility of ringworm infection.

CHARACTERISTICS An ultraviolet light is held over the animal's coat. If areas of apple-green fluorescence are seen, the possibility of ringworm exists and a culture should be taken.

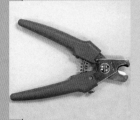

CHAPTER 3

Instruments for Small and Exotic Animals

These instruments are used when caring for and treating small animals.

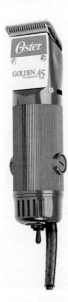

Animal Clippers

All species

FUNCTION To run the clipper blades that shave the hair from an animal's skin.

COMMON NAME Clippers

CHARACTERISTICS This electric clipper has detachable blades that allow the user to shave the hair all the way down to the skin or just to shorten it.

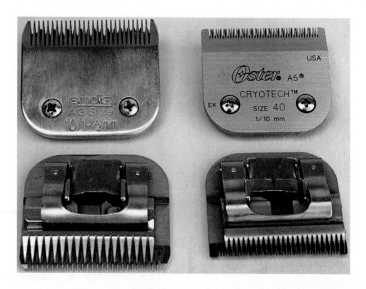

Clipper Blades

All species

FUNCTION To shave the hair from an animal's skin.

CHARACTERISTICS Blades of varying lengths either remove the hair completely or leave the hair as long as 2 to 4 inches. The blades most commonly used in veterinary medicine are the number 40 blade, which removes all the hair for the purpose of surgical preparation and for venipunctures, and the number 10 blade, which leaves approximately ¼ inch of hair and is used to remove matted hair from long-haired animals.

CAUTION
Using a blade with missing teeth or tipping the blade up too far on the animal can cause painful gouges in the skin.

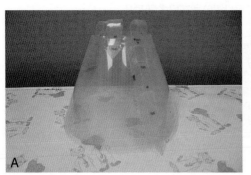 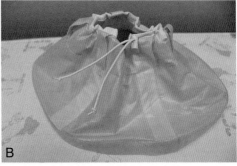

Elizabethan Collar (A) and Soft E Collar (B)

Small animal species

FUNCTION To prevent self-mutilation and bandage destruction.

COMMON NAME E collar

CHARACTERISTICS A cone-shaped collar is custom fitted to the animal. It is important to ensure that the animal's muzzle does not extend past the edge of the collar and that the collar is big enough to fit comfortably around the animal's neck without causing choking. Care must be taken to raise food and water receptacles to a level the animal can reach with the traditional plastic E collar. The soft E collars are used when an animal just cannot tolerate the hard-sided collar. They can reach food and water more easily and do not damage furniture or people if they run into them!

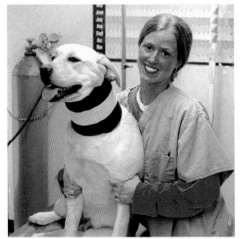

Foam Neck Collar

JorVet Air Bumper Collar

Collar—Neck—Foam Collars and JorVet Air Bumper

Small animal species

FUNCTION To prevent self-mutilation and bandage destruction and to prevent movement of the neck when it has been injured.

CHARACTERISTICS These tight-fitting collars encircle the entire length of the neck. It is important to ensure that they have been properly fitted (neither too long nor too short) and that the animal can reach its food and water. The air bumper collar is inflated to fit around the animal's neck. The foam collar is held together with adhesive tape.

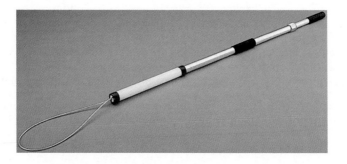

Dog Snare or Capture Pole

Small animal species

FUNCTION To capture and secure the head of an animal so that it may be placed in a cage or run or injected with a sedative.

CHARACTERISTICS The snare or pole is made of aluminum and has a nylon-coated cable that forms a noose. The noose can be lengthened or shortened as needed so that it slips over the head of the animal. The noose can be tightened around the neck to maintain control of the head. Most poles have a stop that prevents inadvertent choking of the animal. Animals should never be lifted off the ground by the snare since that can cause damage to the muscles of the neck or disarticulation of the vertebrae.

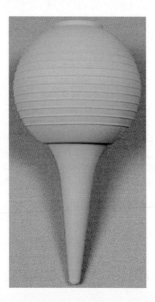

Ear Bulb Syringe

All species

FUNCTION To deliver cleansing solutions to the ear canal. It can also be used to flush wounds.

COMMON NAME Bulb syringe

CHARACTERISTICS A rubber bulb ends in a tapered tube that can be inserted into the ear canal or into a wound. It can also be used to suction the nares or oral cavity in newborns. Squeezing the bulb then releasing it draws solution into the bulb; squeezing again delivers the solution.

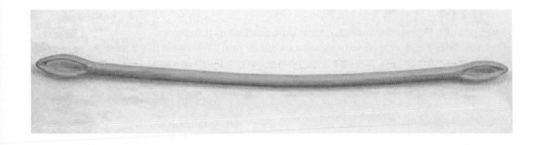

Fecal Loop

All species

FUNCTION To retrieve a sample of feces from the rectum.

CHARACTERISTICS A long plastic shaft ends in a loop at each end. The end is lubricated and gently inserted into the rectum, where the loop gathers any fecal material present. This allows a fecal test to be run without waiting for nature's call. The standard loop is 3⁄8 x 9 inches long; the puppy/kitten loop is 1⁄4 × 43⁄4 inches long.

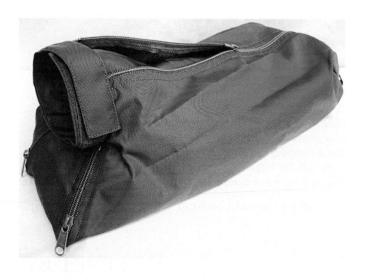

Feline Restraint Bag

Small animal species

FUNCTION To hold a fractious cat securely while a procedure is being performed.

COMMON NAME Cat bag

CHARACTERISTICS A bag into which a cat can be placed to control movement of the head and legs. Zippers allow access to the legs for venipunctures and injections. Medications can be administered to the eyes, ears, and mouth.

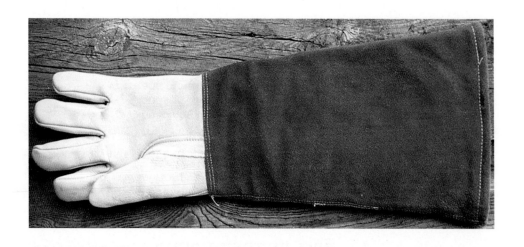

Gauntlets—Restraint Gloves

Small animal and exotic species

FUNCTION To protect the handler from severe scratches and some bites.

CHARACTERISTICS Heavy leather gloves come with extended armbands that protect the handler's hands and forearms when handling fractious animals. These gloves or gauntlets do not keep teeth from penetrating the skin, but they do give the handler some time to get his or her hands clear before the teeth have a chance to penetrate the glove. Care must be taken when holding an animal while wearing gauntlets because tactile sensation is decreased, and inadvertent strangulation may occur.

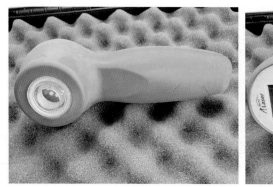
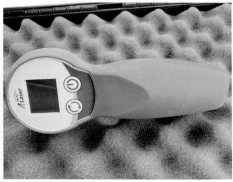

Laser—"My Pet Laser by Multi Radiance Super Pulse Lasers"

All species

FUNCTION Increase vasodilation, bring oxygen, fuel molecules, and other metabolites to injured tissues to aid natural healing.

COMMON NAME Laser

CHARACTERISTICS This handheld laser has multiple settings to adjust the wavelength and depth for individualized treatment of hot spots, lick granulomas, osteoarthritis, general pain, tendinitis, and acute injuries.

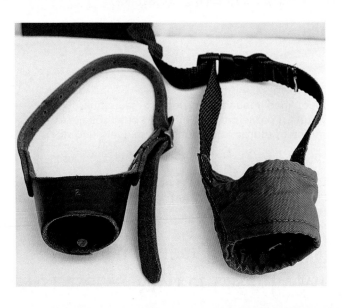

Muzzles—Leather or Nylon

Small animal species

FUNCTION To prevent an animal from biting the handler.

CHARACTERISTICS A tight-fitting strap or a cage-like apparatus is placed around the entire muzzle of the animal. The muzzle must be fitted properly on each animal. If it is not, the likelihood of the animal removing the muzzle or biting through it increases. Muzzles are made to fit cats, dogs, and ferrets.

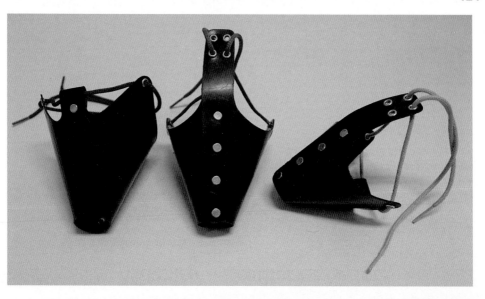

Muzzles—Cone Shaped

Small animal species

FUNCTION Keeps cats and small dogs from being able to bite.

CHARACTERISTICS The cone-shaped muzzle easily slips over a cat or small dog's head and is secured by tying laces around the back of the head. The cone shades the animal's eyes and allows easy breathing from the end of the cone.

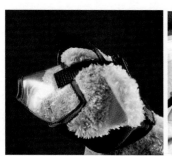 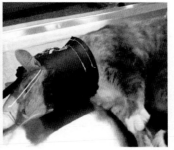 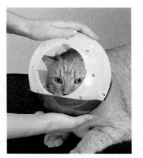

Purr Muzzle

Restraint Air Muzzle

Muzzles—Purr-Muzzle (JorVet) and Restraint Air Muzzle II (Smart Practice)

FUNCTION These muzzles easily slip over the cat's head and are strapped around the neck. They do not block access to the oral cavity and therefore, do not restrict breathing. They cannot be easily removed by the cat using their front legs.

CHARACTERISTICS The transparent cone or ball does not block the cat's vision thus calming the cat better than conventional muzzles. The oral cavity can be evaluated, the jugular vein accessed, and assessment of the eyes is possible with these open-air muzzles.

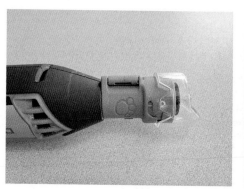
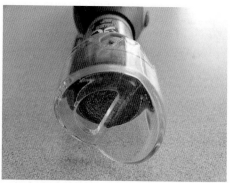

Nail Trimmer—Dremel Pet Grooming Nail Guard

Small animal species

FUNCTION An attachment to a Dremel tool to trim canine toenails.

COMMON NAME Dremel nail trimmer

CHARACTERISTICS This rotary tool attachment will connect to eight different Dremel models with three guard positions to give the correct trimming angle. It also has a dust and fur guard. It significantly speeds up the nail trimming process; however, some dogs have to be conditioned to the noise of the tool itself.

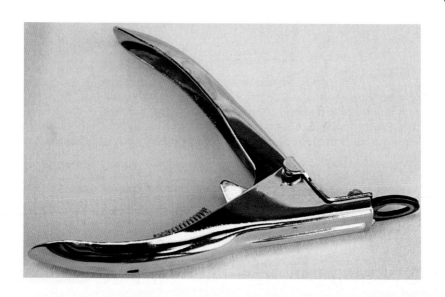

Nail Trimmer—Guillotine

Small animal species

FUNCTION To trim the toenails of small animals.

COMMON NAME Resco

CHARACTERISTICS A guillotine-like blade slides to slice the nail as the handles are squeezed. Care must be taken to hold the trimmer parallel to the pad, so the nail is not cut too short.

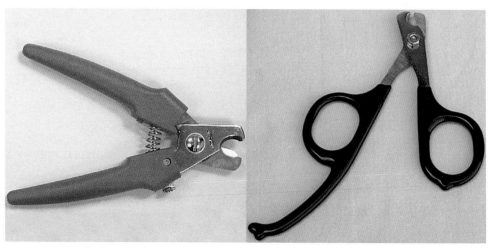

Large nail scissor   Small nail scissor

Nail Trimmer—Scissors

Small animal and exotic species

FUNCTION To trim the toenails of small animals.

COMMON NAME Nail trimmer

CHARACTERISTICS This trimmer is designed much like the White nail trimmer, except that the handles are more substantial on the larger scissors. The trimmers come in a wide variety of sizes, from very small for birds and cats to very large for big dogs.

NOTE
Many have a blade-depth guide that swings over the hole to prevent the operator from removing too much toenail at a time.

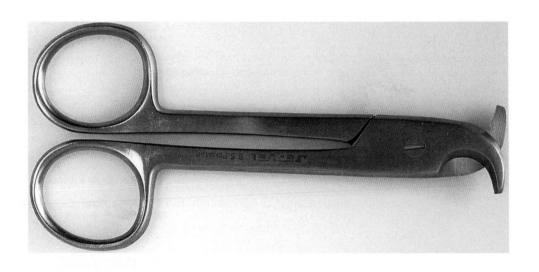

Nail Trimmer—White

Small animal species

FUNCTION To trim a small animal's toenails when they have curved around to the extent of being nearly circular.

COMMON NAME White's

CHARACTERISTICS This scissor-like instrument has jaws that are bowed so that it can accommodate the circular nail. It is most often used when a toenail has grown in a complete circle and close to or into the foot pad.

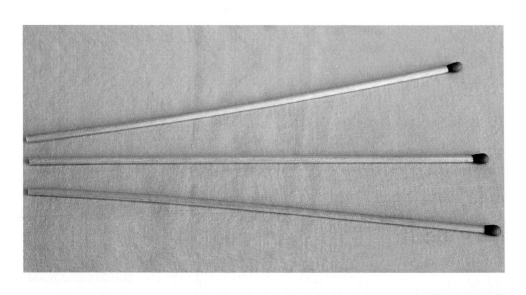

Silver Nitrate Stick

All species

FUNCTION To stop bleeding from blood vessels.

CHARACTERISTICS A small shell of silver nitrate is affixed to a wooden applicator stick. The silver nitrate is applied directly to small blood vessels to cauterize them; this stops the bleeding. Care should be taken not to get wet silver nitrate on skin or clothes because it stains.

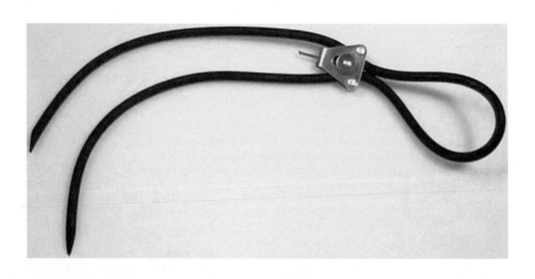

Tourniquet

All species

FUNCTION To occlude a blood vessel so a venipuncture can be performed. It can also be used as a temporary muzzle.

CHARACTERISTICS A rubber or nylon tube is held together by a clip. The tourniquet is tightened around the leg or muzzle by pulling on one end of the tube. It is released by pulling on the clip.

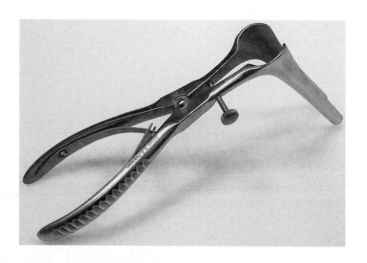

Vaginal Speculum—Killian

FUNCTION To hold open the labia so the vaginal vault can be viewed, swabs taken, and medication delivered to the uterus. It can also be used during the urinary catheterization of a female animal.

CHARACTERISTICS Tapering jaws can be opened by squeezing the handles. A screw set at the top of the handles is turned to keep the jaws open.

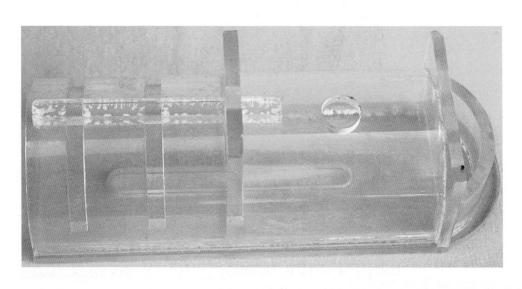

Mouse- and Rat-Restraint Chambers

Exotic animal species

FUNCTION To hold a mouse or rat securely so that a parenteral injection may be administered.

CHARACTERISTICS This plastic tube is equipped with numerous holes and slots that allow access to most body parts for intravenous, subcutaneous, and intramuscular injections. The difficulty involved with this chamber is getting the rodent into it.

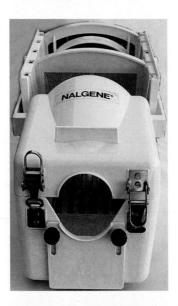

Rabbit-Bleeding Box

Exotic animal species

FUNCTION To hold a rabbit securely for venipuncture to be performed on the ear.

CHARACTERISTICS Usually made of plastic, this box is equipped with a head gate that can be adjusted to fit securely around the rabbit's neck and a tail gate that squeezes the rabbit in tightly so it cannot kick and possibly break its back. The top panel opens wide to allow easy insertion of the rabbit. The floor is grated to enable easy cleanup.

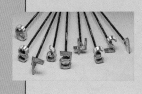

CHAPTER 4

Instruments for the Identification of Animals

These instruments provide the user with a means of permanently or temporarily identifying animals.

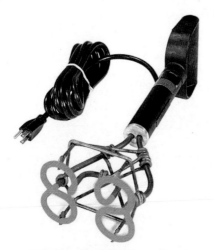

Custom Electric Branding Iron

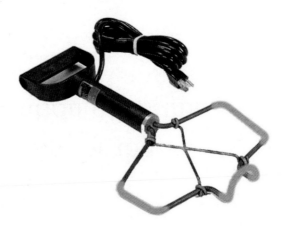

Universal Electric Branding Iron

Branding Irons—Electric

Large animal species

FUNCTION To identify an animal permanently by placing numbers, letters, or designs on the animal's shoulder or hip.

COMMON NAME Electric brander

CHARACTERISTICS This iron has its own heating element in the handle. The brand can be single numbers, letters, or designs, or it can be a series of bends and curves that, when used together, form numbers, letters, or designs. The disadvantage of these irons is that a power source is necessary.

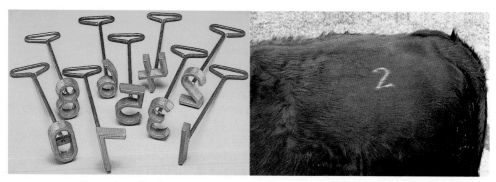

Freeze branding iron

Freeze brand showing pigment loss

Branding Irons—Freeze

Large animal species

FUNCTION   To identify an animal permanently by placing numbers, letters, or designs on the animal's shoulder or hip.

COMMON NAME   Freeze brander

CHARACTERISTICS   These irons are supercooled by liquid nitrogen or a combination of dry ice and alcohol. The irons are placed on the animal's hide, and they kill the pigment-producing cells. The returning hair growth is white, making the mark permanent. The only disadvantage of this method is that it takes approximately 3 months for the hair to grow back.

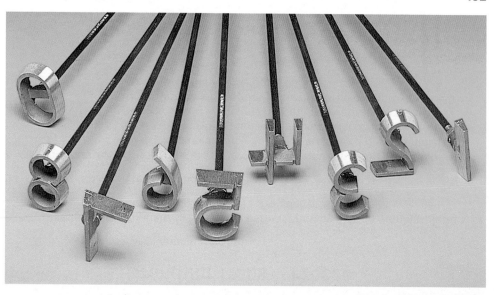

Branding Irons—Hot

Large animal species

FUNCTION   To identify an animal permanently by placing numbers, letters, or designs on the animal's shoulder or hip.

COMMON NAME   Branding irons

CHARACTERISTICS   These irons are made of heavy-duty copper and are available in letters, numbers, and custom designs. The handles are 32 inches long. The irons are heated in a propane heater until they are red hot. The iron is quickly placed against the skin in the body area registered for that particular herd. The iron is held in place until the operator is sure that the skin has been burned. The resulting scar is a permanent mark.

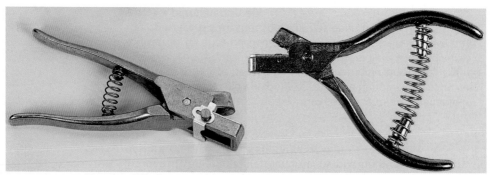

Round and Wedge, to explain whether they are clippers, taggers etc.

Ear Notcher

All species

FUNCTION To make permanent identifying marks on the ears of pigs, goats, and sheep. There are smaller-sized notchers for laboratory animals and exotic animals.

CHARACTERISTICS One jaw of this instrument has a sharp blade that punches a hole or makes a notch; the other is a solid block. The pinna is placed between the jaws of the notcher. When it is squeezed, a piece of tissue is removed from the pinna. The resulting hole or notch is placed around the edge of the pinna and indicates a particular number based on the position and left or right ear. The size of the notch at its base varies from 5/16 to 1/2 inch. A notch of 13/16 can be a V, an inverted U, or a round hole.

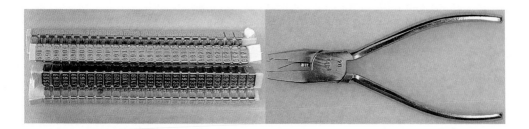

Ear Tag—Hauptner Mouse—Tag and Applicator Laboratory Animal Species

FUNCTION To identify a particular rodent with a numbered tag.

CHARACTERISTICS A small tag bearing an identification number is attached to the ear of a mouse or rat when the handles of the applicator are squeezed.

Universal Total Tagger

Visual Tag – Tamper proof

Visual & FDX EID Tag

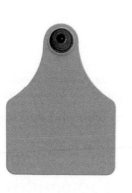

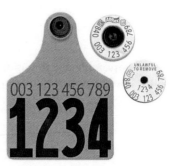

Ear Tags and Applicator

Large animal species

FUNCTION The tags are used to identify individual animals within a herd or flock. The applicator is used to apply ear tags to cattle, sheep, goats, and pigs.

CHARACTERISTICS Visual tags allow the handlers to identify livestock using a combination of numbers and/or letters. The visual and electronic tags work the same way but a scanner can be used to identify the animal via the button applied at the same time. Applicators have a puncturing device onto which the tag is threaded; the other jaw of the applicator is fitted with the back of the tag (much like a human's poststyle pierced earring). The applicator jaws are placed onto the ear, the handles are squeezed and the tag is affixed to the ear. The tag is placed into the ear so that it faces forward. This can be a permanent form of identification but the tags can be cut off or ripped from the ear.

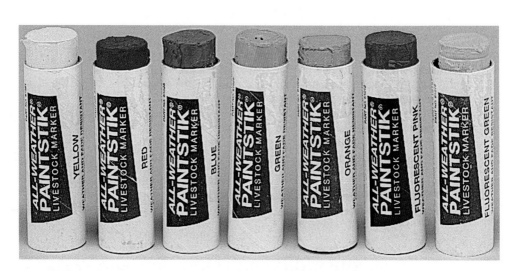

Marking Paint

Large animal species

FUNCTION To mark an animal temporarily.

COMMON NAME Paint stick

CHARACTERISTICS These biodegradable, nontoxic products are designed to be applied to an animal as it is being medicated, vaccinated, or otherwise processed, so as to prevent duplicate administrations. The paints wash or wear off over time. They are available in aerosol sprays, liquid paints, and paint sticks. There is even a paintball gun that can be used to mark an individual in a pasture or a large group without getting near the animal.

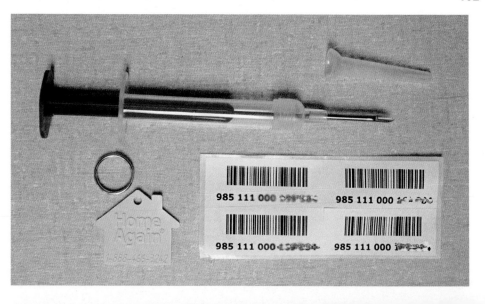

985 111 000

985 111 000

985 111 000

985 111 000

INSTRUMENT Microchip Kit—Small and Large Animal Species

FUNCTION This kit includes the device used to insert an identification microchip into a pet, a chip, and a tag with the same number as the chip.

CHARACTERISTICS This large-bore needle and syringe–like instrument comes loaded with a microchip that has a unique number. The chip is commonly placed under the skin of small animals, directly over the shoulder blades on the top line of the animal. It is often placed inside the lip of large animals. It is important to pinch the insertion point as the needle is being withdrawn because on occasion the microchip is dragged out. Pinching over the hole ensures the microchip stays under the skin.

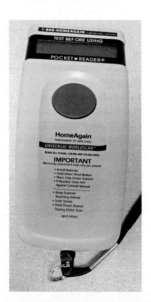

Microchip Reader

Small and large animal species

FUNCTION This device verifies the placement of a microchip under the skin of a pet.

CHARACTERISTICS The microchip reader is used to find and read the microchip under the skin. It can be specific to a particular brand of microchip or it can be a universal one that will read almost all microchips. It is used by pressing and holding down the large button as it is passed over the animal, starting at the shoulders and then down both legs and under the chest, then over the back and down and around the abdomen. The chip tends to migrate and can be found anywhere in the body! If a chip is found, it will beep and display the number and brand.

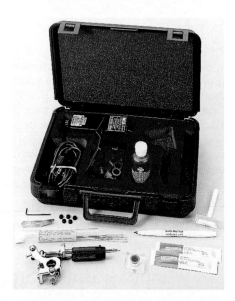

Tattoo Outfit—Electric

All species

FUNCTION To identify an animal permanently by placing numbers, letters, or designs inside the ear, lip, or thigh.

CHARACTERISTICS This outfit operates much like a pen. It has a small motor that moves a needle up and down; the needle is used to puncture the skin in any manner the operator wishes. The ink is applied as the punctures are made or in some models after the punctures are made.

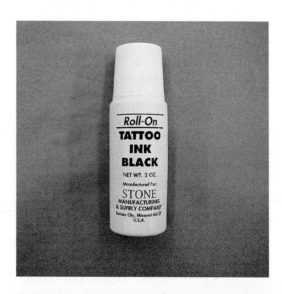

Tattoo Outfit—Ink

All species

FUNCTION To be used with the tattoo outfit to make the punctures permanently visible.

CHARACTERISTICS This indelible ink is placed on the puncture site. The punctures are made, and more ink is applied by the operator using a finger or a soft brush. The ink has to be worked into the punctures; otherwise, it will fade. The ink is available in paste or in liquid form in a roller bottle. The colors available are black, red, green, and white.

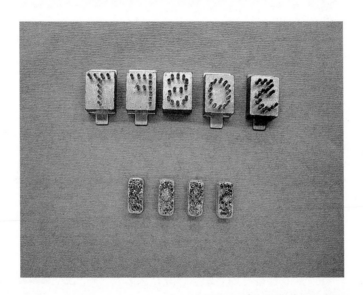

Tattoo Outfit—Letters and Digits

Large animal species

FUNCTION To be used with the tattoo outfit to make punctures for permanent identification.

CHARACTERISTICS Each letter or digit is outlined with sharp spikes on a metal block. The blocks are placed on the jaw of the tattoo outfit and are secured in place by a gate. The letters and digits come in a variety of sizes, from 3/8 inch for large animals to 5/16 and 1/4 inch for small animals.

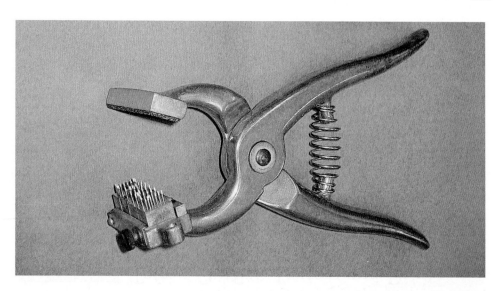

Tattoo Outfit—Manual

Large animal species

FUNCTION To identify an animal permanently by placing numbers or letters inside the ear, lip, or thigh.

CHARACTERISTICS One jaw of the instrument is designed to hold three to five digits or letters; the other has a padded block. The body part is placed between the jaws of the instrument, and the handles are squeezed with enough pressure to puncture the skin. Tattoo ink is then rubbed into the resulting holes. Large- and small-animal tattoo outfits are available. Reasons for tattooing include verification of brucellosis vaccination and identification of a specific purebred animal.

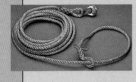

CHAPTER 5

Instruments Used for Bovines

This group of instruments is used to restrain, treat, and care for cattle.

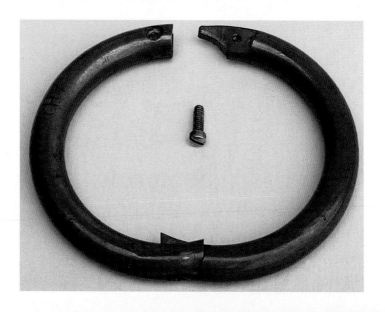

Bull Ring

FUNCTION To control the head of a bull by applying pressure to the nasal septum on a semipermanent basis.

COMMON NAME Nose ring

CHARACTERISTICS The ring is surgically placed in the nasal septum. As the tissue heals, the ring must be turned continually to prevent the tissue from adhering to the ring. Once healing has taken place, staffs with clips on one end are attached to the ring and with the aid of a halter, the bull is led around "by the nose." The rings are available in brass or polished steel. When the bull is no longer of service, the ring can be removed before the animal goes to market.

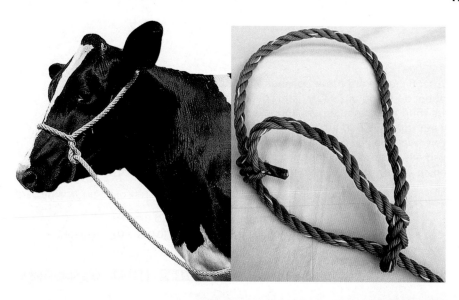

Halter—Adjustable Rope

FUNCTION To control an animal's head while the animal is in a chute or while it is being led.

CHARACTERISTICS This is an adjustable halter. The headstall can be lengthened, and the noseband made wider by pulling the lead rope through a series of loops. The noseband is tightened by pulling on the lead rope. This is an important distinction because, if the noseband is placed around the animal's neck, it can become a choking hazard; in addition, it does not provide good control of the head. When the halter is placed on the head properly, the end of the lead rope should be on the left side of the animal's cheek. These halters are made of round plastic, polyethylene, nylon, or sisal ropes. They come in sizes that fit adults and calves and are used for routine work, such as jugular venipuncture, drenching, surgical procedures on the head, and teaching a show animal how to walk on a lead.

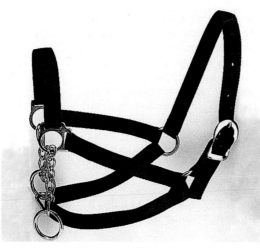

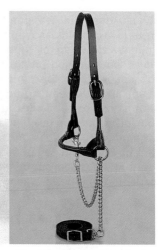

Show halter without lead

Show halter with chain shank

Halter—Fabric Show

FUNCTION To lead cattle in a show.

CHARACTERISTICS The headstall and noseband are held in place by a chain shank that is slipped under the chin and attached to the bottom of the noseband. The chain shank allows better control of an animal than does a nylon strap. This kind of halter is used only after an animal has been taught to be led using a rope halter.

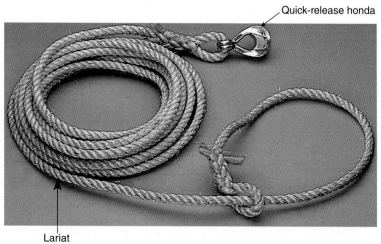

Quick-release honda

Lariat

Lariat With Quick-Release Honda

FUNCTION To capture an animal by the neck or feet.

COMMON NAME Lariat

CHARACTERISTICS Lariats are nylon, nylon-polyester blend, or silk sisal ropes that are between 30 and 35 feet in length. They end in a honda (burner), a Turk's head knot, or a quick-release honda, which holds the loop open. The quick-release honda is a metal device; once the animal has been caught and secured, the loop can be opened by releasing the clasp that holds it together. The honda and the Turk's head knot have to be pulled along the rope for the loop to be opened.

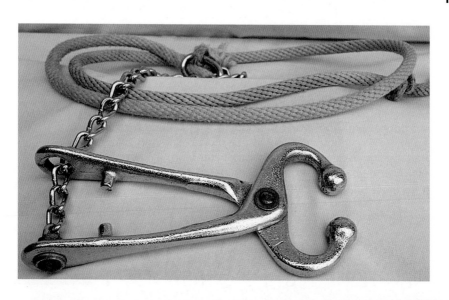

Nose Lead

FUNCTION To control the head by applying pressure to the nasal septum.

COMMON NAME Nose tongs, bull lead, humbug (Canada)

CHARACTERISTICS Two rounded, smooth balls are situated on curved handles. The balls are placed on either side of the nasal septum and the handles are brought together by a rope or chain and secured to a chute or stanchion. The maximum time for application of this instrument is 20 to 30 minutes; after that, the septum loses feeling and the cow struggles. The balls should be inspected for protrusions, which can cause cuts in the nasal septum. If the balls are too close together, the circulation is cut off faster. If they are too far apart, the instrument slips off.

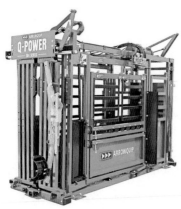

Hydraulic chute

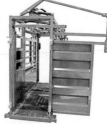

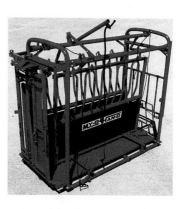

Manual chute

Squeeze Chute—Hydraulic and Manual

FUNCTION To secure a cow or bull in place while maintaining access to its head, feet, and rear.

COMMON NAME Chute

CHARACTERISTICS Most chutes work on the principle of catching the head with some type of squeeze mechanism. Lateral movement is prevented by squeezing the walls of the chute together. Access to the rear is facilitated by a gate or bar that is placed across the back legs of the animal. Feet can be examined by lowering the side panels. This is an extremely useful instrument for cattle restraint, especially for beef cattle. The hydraulic chute is an advancement in safety. Instead of pulling or pushing levers to capture a cow, a push of the buttons will operate the chute quickly and efficiently.

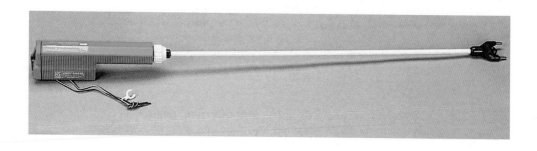

Cattle Prods

FUNCTION To make livestock move into chutes or alleyways.

COMMON NAME Hot shot

CHARACTERISTICS These prods are battery powered so they can deliver an electric jolt to an animal. Proper placement is important. To move an animal forward rather than down, the electrodes should be placed under the tail or anywhere on the vertical surface of the rump. An animal can be turned, if the prod is used on the side of the body or the neck. If the electrodes are placed on the top of the body, the animal becomes confused because the only way for it to move is down. This is a fairly rough form of motivation and should be used judiciously.

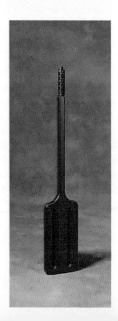

Livestock Sorting Paddle or Cattle Paddle

FUNCTION The hard plastic paddle is utilized to move cattle along or to make the handler look bigger by extending their arms.

CHARACTERISTICS

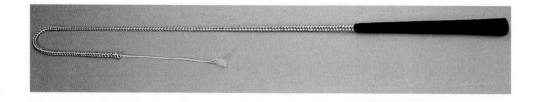

Whips

FUNCTION To make livestock move and to make the handler look bigger.

CHARACTERISTICS A fiberglass shaft ends in a nylon popper that can be flicked at an animal that is balking or refusing to move. The ideal areas to aim for are the heels or across the buttocks; that makes the animal move forward. The whip can also be extended out to the side of the handler to make it look as though the handler has long arms, which is useful in getting an animal to turn or move past. Whips have poppers of varying lengths: a driving whip has a 7-inch popper; a lunge whip, which is used for horses, has a 6-foot popper; and a classic stock whip has a popper that is between 8 and 18 inches long. Some herders tie a small leather strap to the popper for an additional popping sound.

194

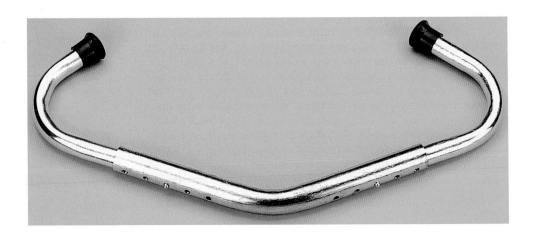

Antikick Bar

FUNCTION To control kicking.

CHARACTERISTICS With push-button adjustments, one end is "hooked" under the flaccid ligament just above the udder and the other end is quickly "hooked" over the top of the spine. This enables optimal control.

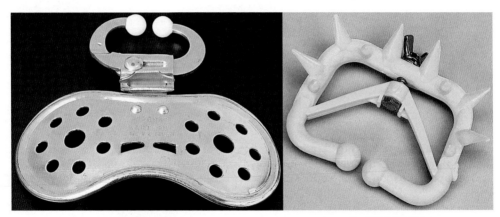

Calf weaner

Kant-Suk weaner

Calf Weaners

FUNCTION To keep weaned calves and adults from nursing.

CHARACTERISTICS This device is attached to the nasal septum of an animal that insists on nursing long after it has been weaned. The device has prongs that prick the udder, making the cow kick the offender, or it has a flap that rests on the nose and prevents the animal from nursing. Both forms allow the animal to eat and drink normally.

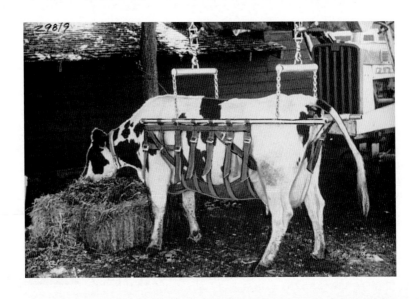

Cow Sling

FUNCTION To get a cow back on its feet after surgery, injury, or illness.

CHARACTERISTICS A series of straps are positioned under the animal's chest, one in front of the front legs and the rest over the rib cage. The sling is brought up the animal's sides and attached to bars that can be attached to crossbeams in the ceiling or to carts for small animals. Models are available for sheep, horses, and dogs.

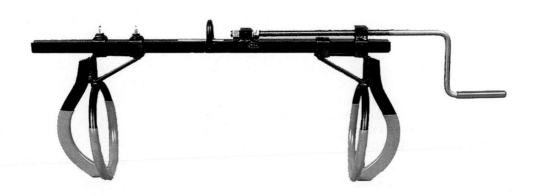

Hip Lift

FUNCTION   To assist a cow to stand; most commonly used in postparturient paresis, milk fever, generalized weakness, obturator paralysis caused by fracture repairs, and when a cow is down on wet cement.

CHARACTERISTICS   Padded rings are attached to a sturdy cross that can be lengthened by turning a crank. The bar is adjusted so that the rings fit tightly to the cow's hips. A cable is attached to the bar and passed over a beam; a winch or a come-a-long is used to hoist up the cow so that it is standing on its feet.

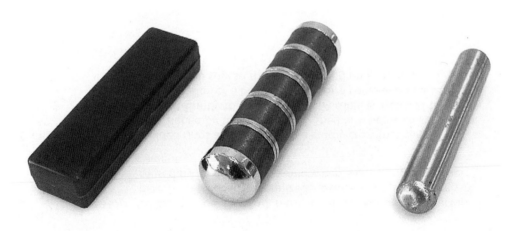

Magnets

FUNCTION To collect and hold metal that has been ingested by cattle as they eat. The metal can cause "hardware disease," if allowed to pass through the rumen.

CHARACTERISTICS Three-inch magnets are passed into the rumen through the mouth. They remain in the rumen and collect bits of wire, nails, and other metal items that are inadvertently swallowed. Unfortunately, this is the only option for cattle as they cannot spit.

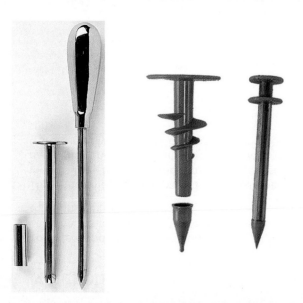

Trocar and Cannula

FUNCTION   To release the rumen gases that cause bloating.

CHARACTERISTICS   A trocar consists of a sharp metal shaft attached to a handle and a cannula that is a hollow tube in which the trocar is placed. A small incision is made in the skin and muscle directly above the rumen. The trocar is plunged into the incision and then the cannula is held in place while the trocar is removed. This allows gases to escape from the rumen. The cannula is left in place until the reason for the bloating has passed, or in cases of chronic bloating, it can be left in place indefinitely.

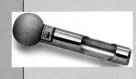

CHAPTER 6

Instruments for Dehorning Animals

This chapter covers instruments used to remove horns from animals.

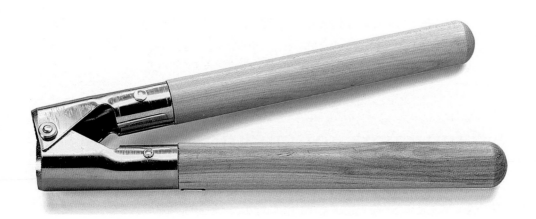

Barnes Dehorner

FUNCTION To remove small horns from calves, goats, and sheep.

CHARACTERISTICS Sharp, half-curved blades are affixed to handles that are 12 to 17½ inches long. The dehorner blades are positioned around the horn with the handles close together. To cut the horn off, the handles are pulled away from each other engaging the blades. This allows the user to place the blades as close to the skull as possible so that the entire horn is removed.

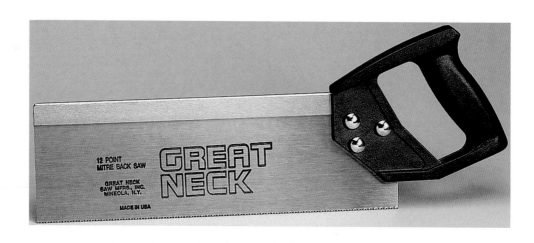

Dehorning Saw

FUNCTION To shorten long, large horns to the level of the head or to smooth a horn that has been broken.

CHARACTERISTICS A square saw blade is attached to a standard saw handle.

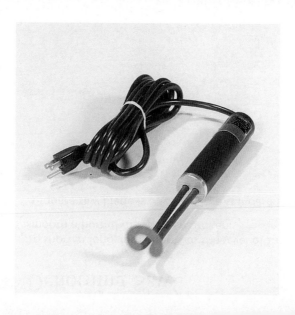

Electric Dehorner

FUNCTION To remove a horn button with high temperature

CHARACTERISTICS This dehorning iron is placed around the base of the horn button and rotated to make sure the entire horn is exposed to the high temperature for a few seconds only. Within 4 to 6 weeks the horn button will drop off leaving a well-healed area.

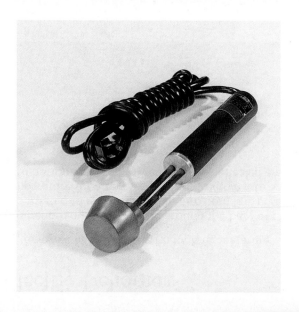

Electric Searing Iron

FUNCTION To sear blood vessels after a horn has been removed. This stops the loss of blood and decreases infection rates.

CHARACTERISTICS The super-hard cast aluminum bronze heats quickly and has lasting durability.

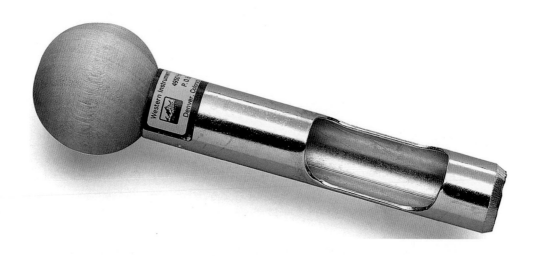

Horn Gouge or Tube Dehorner

FUNCTION To remove horn buds or very small horns.

CHARACTERISTICS A metal tube ending with a very sharp edge is used to cut through tissue; the handle is usually rounded for easy gripping. The tube is pushed down around the horn until it hits the skull, then twisted around, first one way and then the other. The instrument is moved to a 45-degree angle to scoop the horn off the head. Another name for this instrument is the tube calf dehorner.

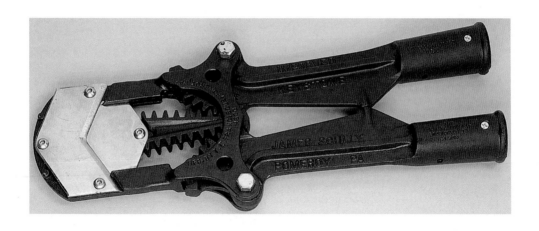

Keystone Dehorner (Guillotine)

FUNCTION To remove medium-sized to large horns.

CHARACTERISTICS This instrument has a blade that slices through the horn much as a guillotine would. When the handles are closed, the blade engages and cuts through the horn. This instrument is very heavy, so only a strong person is capable of operating it.

NOTE
Long wooden handles are placed in the receptacles on the dehorner. They are not shown here.

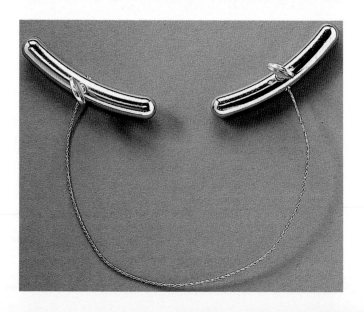

INSTRUMENT# Wire Saw With Handles

FUNCTION To remove large horns.

CHARACTERISTICS A rough-surfaced wire with handles is pulled back and forth across the surface of the horn, and it cuts through the horn.

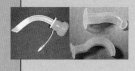

CHAPTER 7

Catheters and Tubes

A variety of tubes and catheters are used in veterinary medicine
to help patients recover from injuries, illnesses, and surgeries.

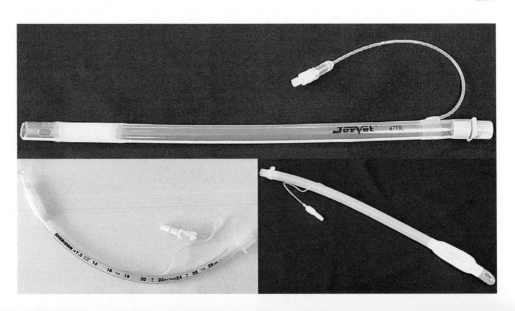

Airway Control—Endotracheal Tube

Small and large animal species

FUNCTION To establish an open airway to deliver gas, anesthesia, or oxygen.

COMMON NAME Trach tube, ET tube

CHARACTERISTICS A flexible tube that is available in a variety of sizes that range from 1- to 14-mm internal diameter for small animals and 16 to 30 mm for large animals. Small animal tubes have a cuff on the end of most tubes, this is used to seal the tracheal opening after insertion of the tube; this prevents the animal from breathing around the tube and prevents fluids from entering the lungs. The cuffs may allow use of a large or small volume of air, which is delivered via a one-way valve attached to the side of the tube. The tubes are made of silicone, polypropylene, or red rubber.

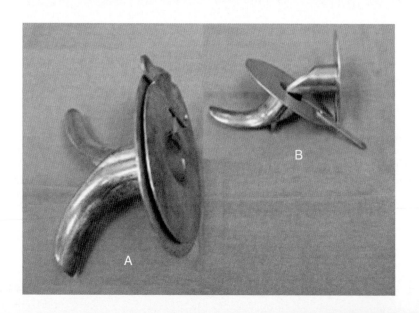

Airway Control—Stainless-Steel Self-Retaining Tracheotomy Tube

Small and large animal species

FUNCTION To establish an airway through the tracheal wall in a patient with an upper airway obstruction or critical illness.

CHARACTERISTICS This stainless-steel tracheotomy tube is utilized in large animals. It has an inside diameter of 22 mm and an outside diameter of 28 mm. It is a two-piece device, an introducer and a Y-shaped "tube" that spreads to hold the device in place.

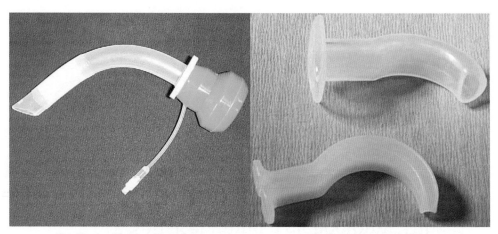

Small animal tracheostomy tube   Equine tracheostomy tube

Airway Control—Tracheostomy Tube

Small and large animal species

FUNCTION To establish an airway through the tracheal wall in a patient with an upper airway obstruction or critical illness.

CHARACTERISTICS A short tube that can be left in place on a short- or long-term basis. It may be cuffed or uncuffed and is made of silicone or silver-plated metal. Sizes range from 2.5- to 3-mm internal diameter for small animals.

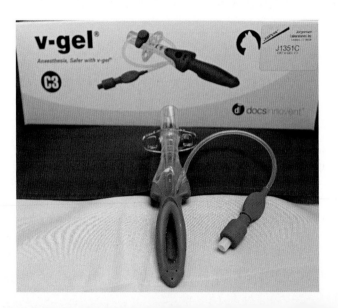

Airway Control—V-Gel Supraglottic Airway

Small animal species

FUNCTION To establish an airway in cats.

CHARACTERISTICS This species-specific airway is anatomically correct to fit securely over and surrounds the epiglottis in cats and rabbits. This is an alternative to intubating a cat with a standard endotracheal tube (ET), which can damage the trachea. There are six sizes for each species. It is reusable, as it can be autoclaved at low temperatures for up to 40 cycles.

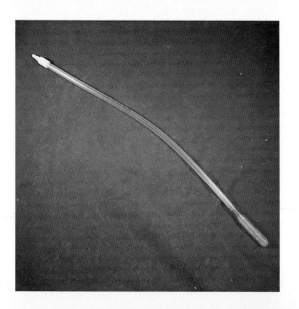

232

INSTRUMENT Esophageal Stethoscope

Small animal species

FUNCTION To allow the heartbeat to be heard; it is useful during procedures that require anesthesia.

CHARACTERISTICS This long flexible tube has a rounded end that is inserted into the esophagus until it rests beneath the heart. The other end is attached to a speaker device that makes the beating of the heart audible. This stethoscope can be used only in animals that have been anesthetized. It comes in a variety of sizes, which are measured by the French (Fr) scale; from the smallest to largest, 12, 18, and 24 Fr are available.

NOTE
It is important to measure with the tube from the tip of the jaw to the heart on the outside of the animal to determine how far to insert the stethoscope.

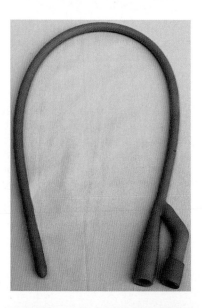

Feeding Tube—Foley Catheter

Small animal species

FUNCTION To catheterize an animal when the catheter must be retained. The catheter can be placed in the esophagus to use as a feeding tube or in the urethra, rectum, or uterus for various reasons.

COMMON NAME Foley

CHARACTERISTICS This soft, silicone-coated, amber latex catheter has a balloon of 3, 5, or 30 mL near the end close to the tapered tip. The balloon is inflated with water or air, and that is used to keep the catheter in place. They come in sizes of 5 to 25 Fr.

Nasogastric feeding tube

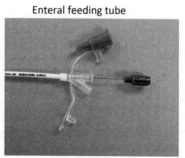

Enteral feeding tube

Enteral feeding tube

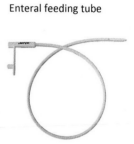

Feeding Tubes—Nasogastric and Enteral

Small and large animal species

FUNCTION A means of providing nutrients over long periods.

CHARACTERISTICS The nasogastric tube is directed through the nasal passages and into the stomach. It can be removed after the nutrition is delivered or left in place for several weeks. The enteral feeding tube is placed into the stomach through the abdominal wall or from the neck. There are many types of nasogastric and enteral feeding tubes for all species of animals.

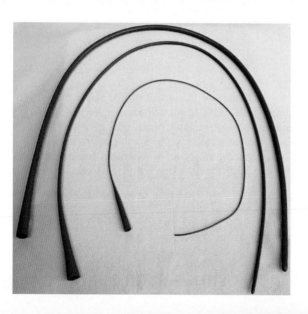

Feeding Tube—Rubber

Small animal species

FUNCTION To be used as a nasogastric or esophageal feeding tube or a urinary catheter.

CHARACTERISTICS This flexible red rubber catheter is approximately 12- to 18-inches long and is available in 8 to 20 Fr, in increments of 2, as well as in 24 and 28 Fr. Most have lateral "eyes" or openings close to the tapering tip.

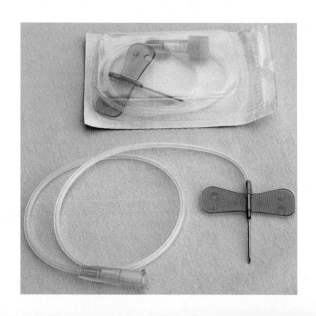

Intravenous Equipment—Butterfly or Winged Infusion Sets

Small and large animal species

FUNCTION To establish a port into a vein to deliver intravenous (IV) fluids or to draw blood samples from very small animals such as rabbits and kittens.

COMMON NAME Butterfly catheter

CHARACTERISTICS This catheter has a standard 1-inch needle that is inserted into a vein. The wings are used to secure the catheter in place. The long tube on this catheter must be filled with fluid before insertion; otherwise, air will be introduced into the vein when the fluids are attached. This catheter is easy to place but difficult to keep in place because of the needle.

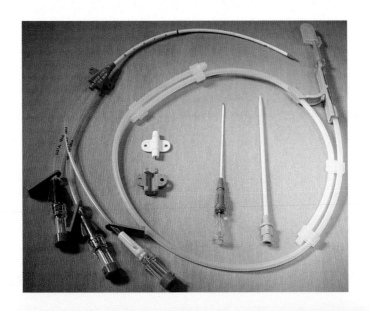

Intravenous Equipment—Central Venous Catheter

Small and large animal species

FUNCTION To establish a port into a vein or artery to deliver IV fluids over an extended period or to monitor central venous pressure or blood pressure by placement in an artery.

COMMON NAME Central line

CHARACTERISTICS This catheter is usually quite long, and several steps are involved in its placement. The advantage of the catheter is that it can be left in place for more than 72 hours if strict attention is paid to sterile conditions during placement. This particular catheter comes with three ports that can accept different medications that may react with each other if given into the same port. This same type of catheter can be used for IV nutritional support; the nutritional type of catheter usually does not have more than one port.

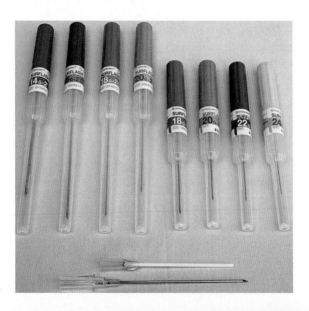

Intravenous Equipment—Indwelling Intravenous Catheter

Small and large animal species

FUNCTION To establish a port into a vein to deliver IV fluids to large and small animals.

COMMON NAME IV catheter

CHARACTERISTICS A flexible catheter is placed over a needle or through a needle. The needle is used to puncture the skin and vessel; the catheter is then threaded into the vein. The needle is removed after the catheter has been placed. The catheter has a standard hub that receives the IV drip set or syringe tip. The hub is also used to secure the catheter to the animal's body. Sizes range from a 24-gauge × ¾ inch to 10-gauge × 5¼ inches. They can be made of polyurethane, Teflon, or Pebax or of nonreactive polyurethane for long-term use.

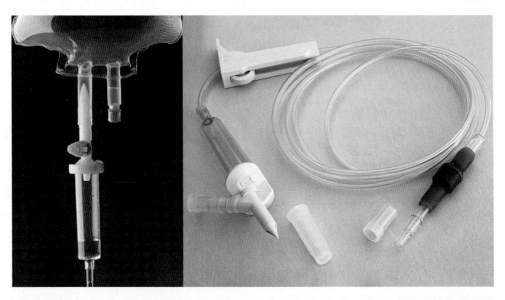

Intravenous Equipment—Drip Sets or IV Drip Sets

Small and large animal species

FUNCTION To provide a connection between the IV catheter and the IV fluids and to regulate the flow of the fluids.

COMMON NAME IV drip set, IV-line, venous sets

CHARACTERISTICS A long flexible tube with various ports and shut-off valves is attached to the reservoir of the IV fluids and then attached to the IV catheter. Drip sets come in a variety of sizes that deliver 10, 15, 20, or 60 drops per minute. It is important to note the size of the drip set in use so the correct amount of fluid can be delivered in the prescribed time.

248

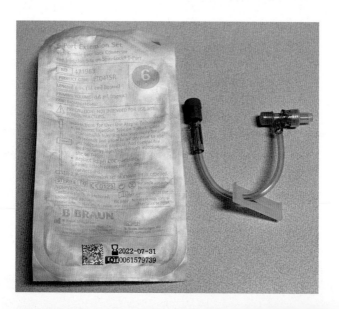

Intravenous Equipment—Extension Port or T-Port

Small and large animal species

FUNCTION Establishes two injection ports into one catheter.

CHARACTERISTICS This extension tube is attached between the IV catheter and IV tube. The side port allows for quick, easy access without fear of dislodging the catheter.

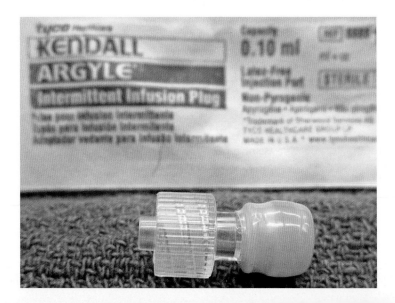

Intravenous Equipment—Injection Cap

Small and large animal species

FUNCTION To close off the end of a catheter.

CHARACTERISTICS A small plastic cap is designed to be inserted into the hub of a catheter. It has a rubber stopper on the other end that can be punctured by a standard hypodermic needle. This allows the IV drip set to be inserted and removed without fear of dislodging the catheter or of introducing bacteria when removing the tubing. It is also used to maintain a catheter's placement.

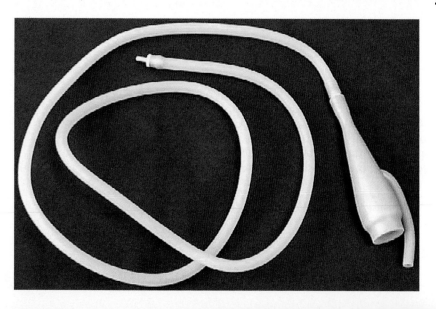

Intravenous Equipment—Simplex Intravenous Bell Sets

Large animal species

FUNCTION To provide a connection between the IV catheter and the IV fluids and to regulate the flow of those fluids.

COMMON NAME Gravity IV set

CHARACTERISTICS This set uses gravity to enable the flow of the fluids. Latex tubing has a flexible funnel at one end that fits over the top of a bottle; the other end of the tubing has a tip that fits into a standard catheter hub. Some models have an air hose that can be clamped to prevent the fluids from flowing. The bottle is raised or lowered to speed up or slow down the rate at which the fluids are introduced into the animal. This set is used in large animals.

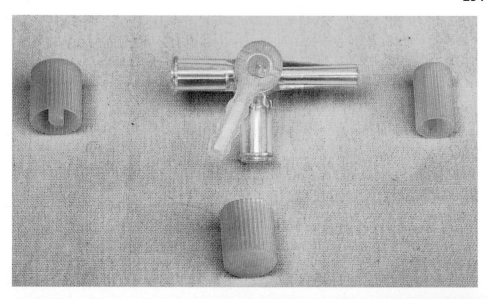

Intravenous Equipment—Three-Way Stopcock

Small and large animal species

FUNCTION To give the user more than one port to administer solutions via syringes or other IV lines.

COMMON NAME Stopcock

CHARACTERISTICS This plastic instrument has a tip that fits into the end of a catheter; the other two ends have standard hubs that accept syringes or IV lines. The dial on the top directs the flow into the catheter from one hub or the other.

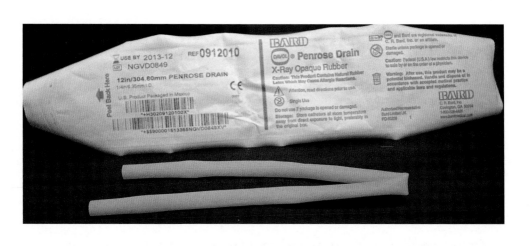

Penrose Drain

All animal species

FUNCTION Provides body fluids with a path to exit the body.

CHARACTERISTICS A flexible rubber tube is placed under the skin of large wounds to allow fluids to evacuate around the tube while the wound heals. It requires daily care to keep the wound draining while the wound heals and to keep the skin clean and protected.

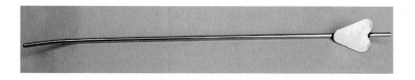

Urinary Catheters—Female Canine Catheter

Small animal species

FUNCTION To catheterize the bladder or uterus of a female dog.

CHARACTERISTICS This stainless-steel catheter is approximately 10-inches long and tapers to a rounded tip. The opposing end has a heart-shaped handle.

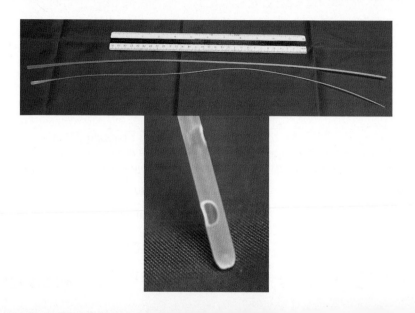

Urethral Catheter—Polypropylene

Small animal species

FUNCTION To catheterize a male dog, in most cases because of urethral blockage but also to secure a urine sample.

COMMON NAME Dog catheter

CHARACTERISTICS A polypropylene catheter approximately 18-inches long tapers to a rounded point. It is available in a range of sizes: 3½, 5, 8, 10, and 14 Fr.

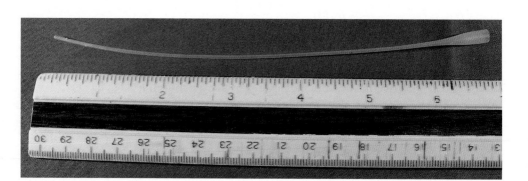

Urinary Catheters—Polypropylene Tom Cat Catheter

Small animal species

FUNCTION To catheterize a male cat, in most cases because of urethral blockage but also to secure a urine sample.

CHARACTERISTICS A polypropylene catheter approximately 6-inches long tapers to a rounded point.

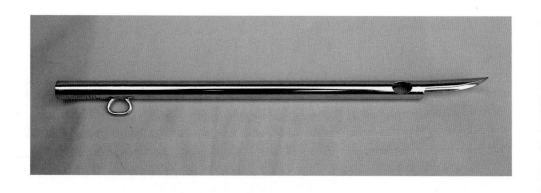

Urinary Catheter—Cow

Large animal species

FUNCTION To catheterize the bladder.

CHARACTERISTICS This stainless-steel catheter has a scooped-out area just before the tip.

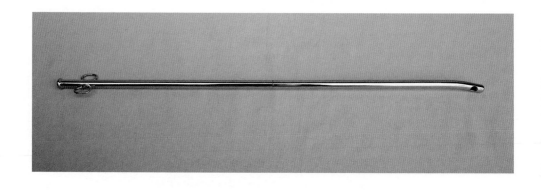

Urinary Catheter—Mare

Large animal species

FUNCTION To catheterize the bladder.

CHARACTERISTICS A slightly angled, stainless-steel tube; it has opposite-facing eyes on the end.

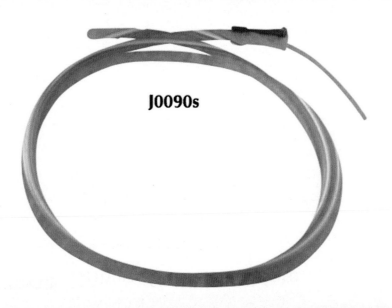

J0090s

Urinary Catheter—Stallion

Large animal species

FUNCTION To catheterize a male horse.

CHARACTERISTICS This flexible catheter is 6.6 mm × 137 cm long.

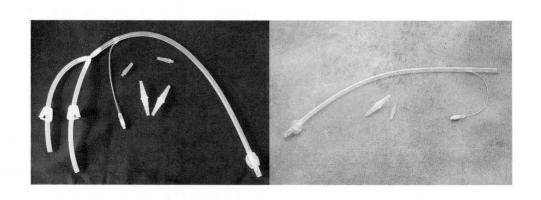

Uterine-Flushing Catheter—Mare

Large animal species

FUNCTION To collect or transfer an embryo or to medicate the uterus.

CHARACTERISTICS This flexible catheter comes in 33 Fr and is 65 or 135 cm in length. It has an inflatable cuff and two different adapters for attaching tubing or a standard Luer fitting.

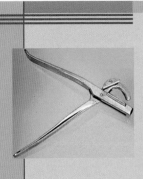

CHAPTER 8

Instruments for Castration of Large Animals

This chapter covers instruments that are used to castrate, tail dock, and ear notch large animals.

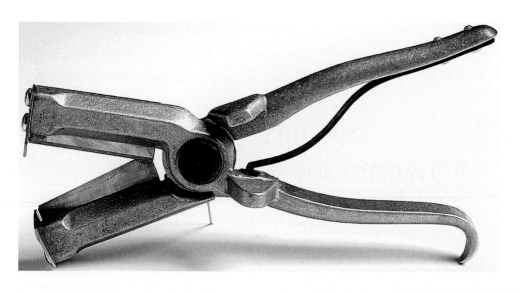

All-in-One Lamb Castrator, Docker, and Ear Marker

FUNCTION To castrate, dock the tails, and notch the ears of lambs, kids, and piglets.

CHARACTERISTICS Sharp blades on the side of the instrument are used to dock the tail and nip off the end of the scrotal sac. The jaws are used to stretch-pull the testicles out of the body. The ear notcher is located at the base of the knife section.

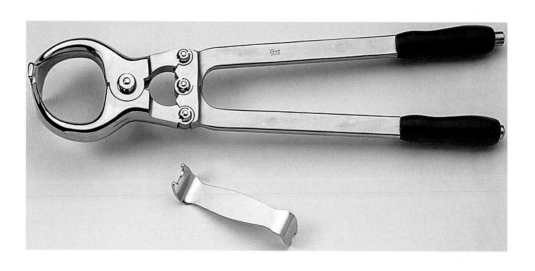

Burdizzo Emasculatome

FUNCTION   To perform a bloodless castration on a large animal.

COMMON NAME   Burdizzo

CHARACTERISTICS   Blunt jaws have a double-action wrenching device, which crushes the blood vessel and spermatic cord inside the skin of the testicle, making it a bloodless castration. This is not recommended on very large testicles because it is difficult to apply enough pressure. This instrument is available in 9-, 12-, 14-, 16-, and 19-inch lengths. A knee brace is available for the larger models.

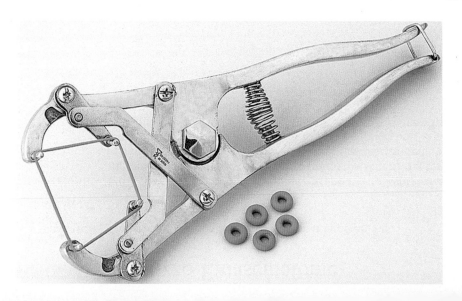

Elastrator

FUNCTION To perform a bloodless castration or tail dock on a large animal.

CHARACTERISTICS This instrument has pegs; a thick rubber band can be placed around them. The handles are squeezed to stretch the rubber band so that it goes around the testicle or tail. The rubber band restricts blood flow to the testicle or tail and is left in place until the testicle or tail falls off. This tool is considered a bloodless technique.

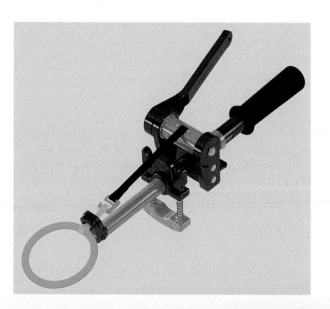

INSTRUMENT # Elastrator and Dehorner—Callicrate PRO Bander

FUNCTION

To remove testicles and horns by applying a rubber band tightly around the tissue.

CHARACTERISTICS

This instrument is designed to assist in correctly placing the rubber band around the scrotum approximately 1 inch above the testicles or at the base of the horn. The ratchet is then engaged until the tightness indicator ring has reached the designated line on the handle. Then the cutter is depressed to cut the band. The band stays in place cutting off the blood supply to these areas until the testicles or horn drops off.

282

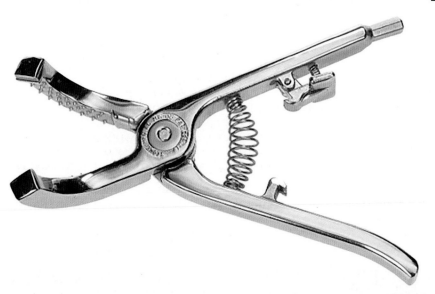

Emasculator—Henderson

FUNCTION Removes testicles by crushing the blood vessels and surrounding tissues, then removal occurs by spinning the testicle with an electric drill.

CHARACTERISTICS The instrument is attached to a cordless drill and then the scrotum is cut with the Newberry castrating knife, which allows the testicles to drop out of the scrotum. The jaws of the instrument are clamped above one of the testicles and locked by squeezing the handles together. The drill is turned on and the testicle is spun until it falls away from the body. The spinning action twists the blood vessels tight and prevents bleeding as well as splitting the tissues.

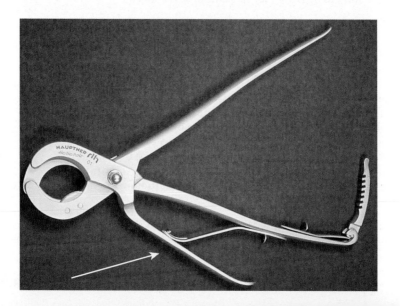

Emasculator—Reimer

FUNCTION To perform a castration on a large animal.

CHARACTERISTICS This instrument has a crushing action that is separate from the cutting lever *(arrow)*. The testicle is surrounded by the jaws. The crushing is done by applying pressure and locking the jaws. The cutting lever is then squeezed to remove the testicle. It is important to ensure that the instrument is positioned so that the crushed tissue is close to the body to prevent hemorrhaging.

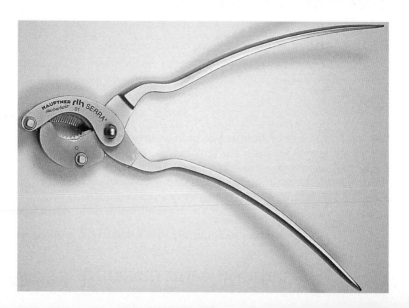

Emasculator—Serra

FUNCTION To perform castration on a large animal.

CHARACTERISTICS This instrument is designed to draw the spermatic cord and blood vessel concentrically into the jaws, which prevents the cords from slipping. In addition, they are pressed together and crushed as they are cut, which prevents postoperative hemorrhaging.

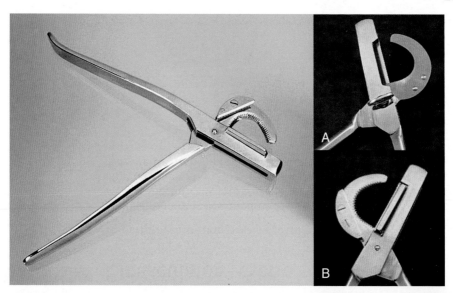

White Emasculator

FUNCTION To perform castration on a large animal.

CHARACTERISTICS This instrument has a crushing platform (A) as well as a cutting blade (B) incorporated into the jaws. The scrotal sac is incised with a scalpel blade; the testicle is pulled out of the scrotum and the emasculator is applied so that the cutting edge is next to the testicle and the crushing platform (A) is toward the body. When the handles are squeezed, the testicle is severed from the body, and the blood vessel and spermatic cord are crushed. This prevents heavy bleeding. If applied incorrectly, the blood vessel is not crushed, which can cause severe hemorrhaging.

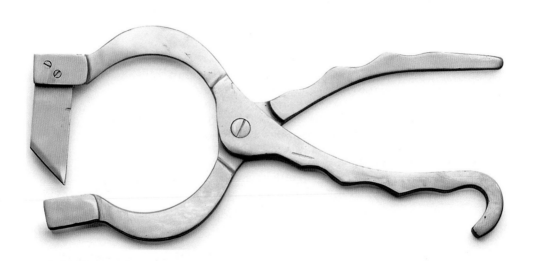

Newberry Castrating Knife

FUNCTION To cut the scrotal sac for testicle exposure.

CHARACTERISTICS A sharp blade is attached to handles; this allows the handler to split the scrotal sac in a controlled manner.

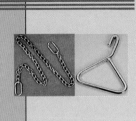

CHAPTER 9

Obstetrical Instruments

This section covers instruments that are used to assist with obstetrical (OB) examinations, dystocia and breeding, or infertility issues.

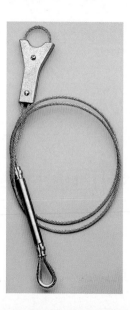

Subcategory—Dystocia Instruments

Calf snare

FUNCTION To assist with the delivery of a calf.

CHARACTERISTICS This nylon-coated cable is equipped with a locking device that will not tighten on the body part to which it is attached. This is very useful in pulling a head into proper alignment and keeping it in place until the calf is delivered.

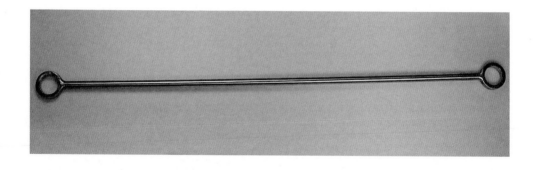

Cornell Detorsion Rod

FUNCTION To correct uterine torsion.

CHARACTERISTICS This instrument has a loop at one end through which a soft rope can be threaded. The resulting loop is attached to the fetus. The other end requires a wooden dowel inserted into the loop to become a handle. The instrument is then turned to undo the uterine torsion.

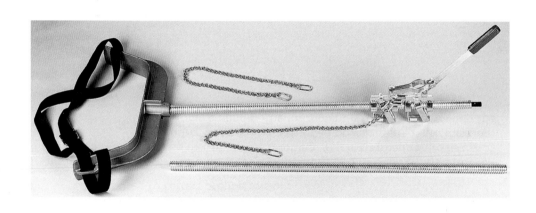

Fetal Extractor

FUNCTION To assist with the delivery of a calf.

COMMON NAME Calf puller, calf jack

CHARACTERISTICS The strap on the brace piece is placed over the hips of the cow. OB chains or straps are attached to the legs of the calf. Along the shaft of the fetal extractor is a come-a-long, which is a cable attached to a ratchet that reels the cable into a spool. The cable is attached to the OB chains, and the user gently inches the calf out of the cow, while working with the cow's contractions and at the correct angles.

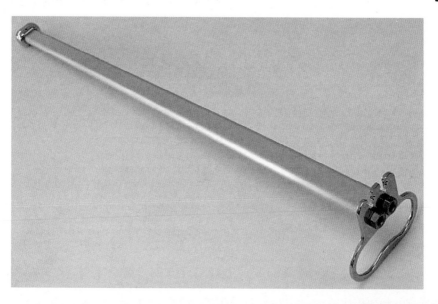

Fetatome

FUNCTION To disarticulate a dead fetus to aid in its removal.

CHARACTERISTICS An OB wire is passed inside the fetatome; it protects the mother's delicate tissues as the saw is worked back and forth.

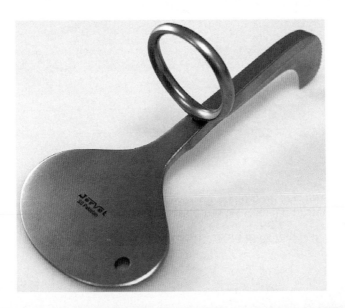

INSTRUMENT   Fetotomy Knife

FUNCTION   To disarticulate a dead fetus to aid in its removal.

CHARACTERISTICS   This instrument is designed to fit into the palm of the hand. The index finger is slipped into the ring and curled over the top of the blade. This allows the knife to be directed to the appropriate area for cutting.

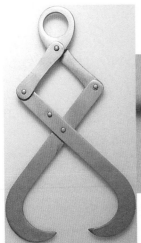

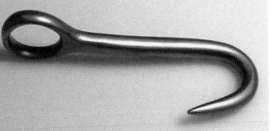

Ostertag's blunt eye hook

Krey OB hook

Krey Obstetrical Hook

FUNCTION To hold onto the fetus while performing an embryotomy.

COMMON NAME OB hook

CHARACTERISTICS The hooks bite into the fetus to hold it steady.

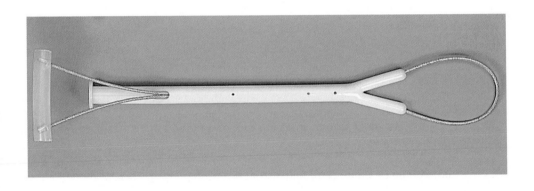

Lambing Extractor

FUNCTION To help a lamb from the birth canal.

CHARACTERISTICS A loop is placed around the lamb's front legs and the body is eased out as the ewe has a contraction.

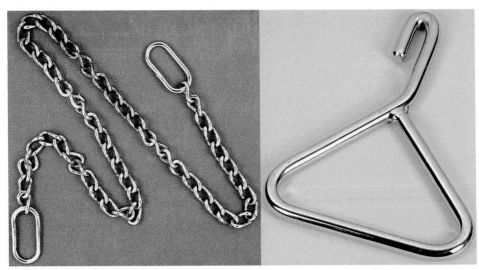

Chains

Handles

Obstetrical Chains and Handles

FUNCTION To assist with the delivery of a calf.

COMMON NAME OB chains and handles

CHARACTERISTICS The chains are flat links that prevent trauma to the calf's legs. The handles have a hook that fits onto the chains at any link for optimal directional and pulling power.

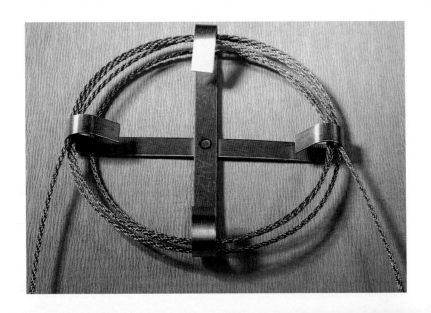

Obstetrical Wire

FUNCTION To disarticulate a dead fetus to aid in its removal.

COMMON NAME OB wire

CHARACTERISTICS This is a rough cable-like material that cuts through bone and sinew when it is rubbed back and forth. As parts are removed, the calf can be pulled from the cow.

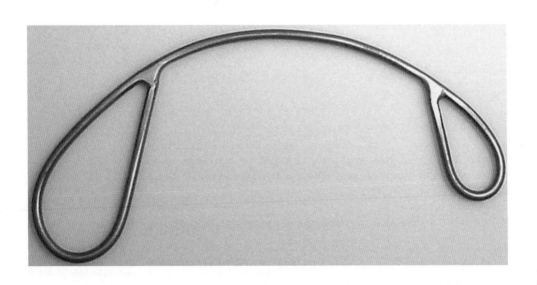

Obstetrical Wire Guide

FUNCTION To help guide the OB wire to the appropriate area for cutting.

CHARACTERISTICS A curved handle ends in a weighted bulb in which the wire is threaded.

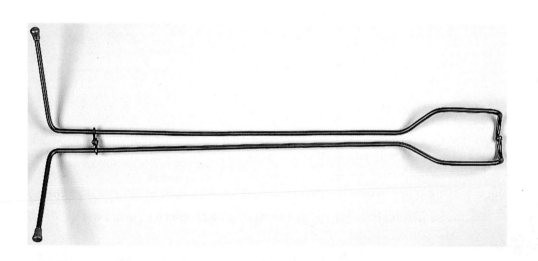

Pig Obstetrical Forceps

FUNCTION To assist in delivering a piglet.

CHARACTERISTICS The hinged, bowed area is designed to open so that it can grasp the head or hips, not the uterine lining.

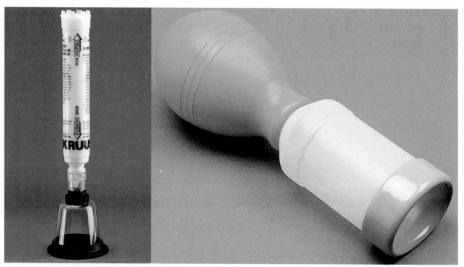

Calf and piglet resuscitator

Lamb resuscitator

Resuscitators for Calf, Foal, Piglet, and Lamb

FUNCTION To provide room air to a large animal newborn that is having difficulty breathing.

CHARACTERISTICS A face mask is designed to fit over the muzzle of the animal; room air is forced into the lungs by bellows or a pump or by breathing into the mouthpiece.

318

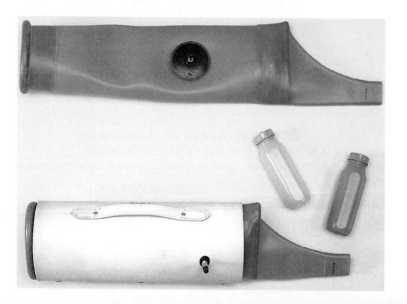

Subcategory—Obstetrical Instruments

Artificial insemination (AI)—artificial vagina

FUNCTION To allow the collection of semen from a stimulated male.

CHARACTERISTICS A hollow tube is fitted with a latex collection liner and is readied for insertion into the penis. Models for cattle, horses, pigs, and sheep are available.

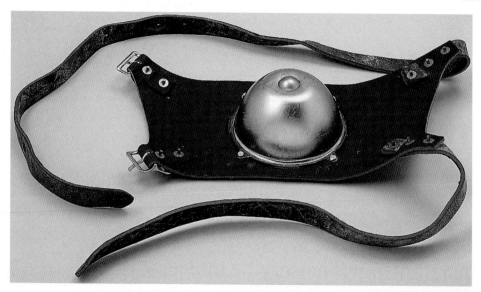

Artificial Insemination—Heat Mount Detector

FUNCTION To mark a cow that is in standing heat.

CHARACTERISTICS A metal reservoir filled with marking paint is attached to a headstall. The headstall is strapped onto a gomer bull so that the reservoir rests under his chin. The reservoir works like an ink pen, marking the cow as the gomer bull slides off her.

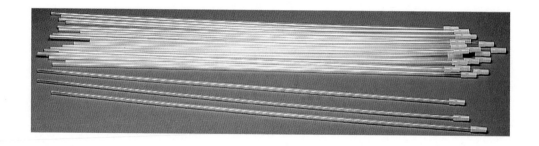

Artificial Insemination—Insemination Pipettes

FUNCTION To deliver semen directly into the uterus.

CHARACTERISTICS These long PVC (polyvinyl chloride) pipettes allow deep insertion so the sperm can be delivered into the uterus.

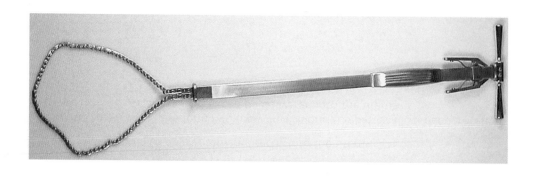

General OB—Ecraseur

FUNCTION To spay a heifer.

CHARACTERISTICS A small incision is made in the side of the animal. The loop is placed around the ovary and facilitates its removal.

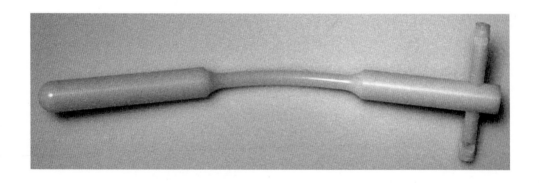

General OB—Freemartin Probe

FUNCTION To check for freemartin heifers and to determine whether a heifer that is a twin to a bull calf has a normal reproductive tract.

CHARACTERISTICS The probe end of this instrument is placed inside the vagina. If it measures 7 cm or less, the heifer is a freemartin. If the heifer is born with a bull twin, the tract may be as large as 14 cm.

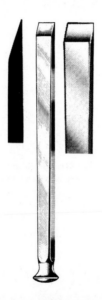

General OB—Pelvic Chisel

FUNCTION To split the uncalcified pubic symphysis so as to widen the pelvic canal, which allows the fetus to be delivered.

CHARACTERISTICS This is a larger version of the orthopedic osteotome. A small incision is made below the ventral commissure of the vulva in the floor of the pelvis. The chisel is placed at the pubic symphysis and struck with a mallet; this widens the birth canal.

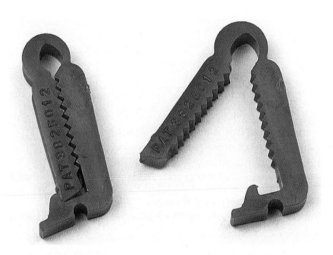

General OB—Umbilical Clamp

FUNCTION To clamp the umbilical cord before it is cut.

CHARACTERISTICS The clamp is made of plastic and has a locking mechanism to keep it in place.

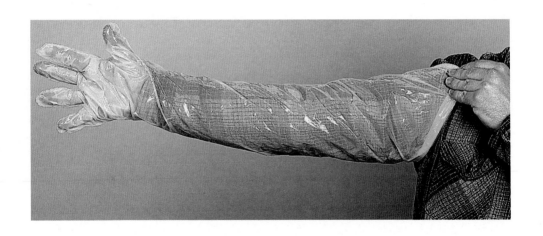

Personal Protection—Obstetrical
Gloves

FUNCTION To protect personnel from zoonotic diseases and keep clothing clean.

CHARACTERISTICS These gloves have extra-long sleeves that reach the shoulders. They are made of plastic or latex and are disposable.

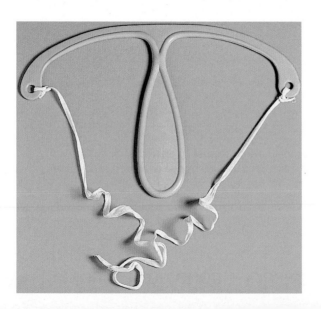

Prolapse Instruments—Ewe Prolapse
Retainer

FUNCTION To retain a vaginal prolapse.

CHARACTERISTICS The paddle is placed inside the vagina and the wings are secured to the outside of the sheep. The retainer does not interfere with lambing and can be left in place for an extended period.

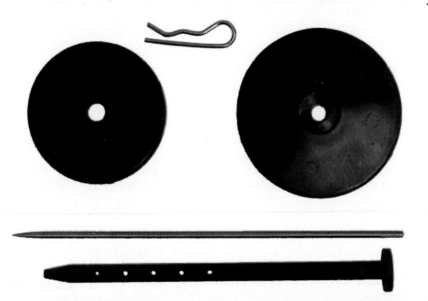

336

Prolapse Instruments—Profix or Johnson Button

FUNCTION Keeps a prolapse from reoccurring.

CHARACTERISTICS Internal fixation of preparturient vaginal prolapse in cattle that allows for normal parturition. The prolapse kit contains a 6-inch plastic trocar, a 3-inch diameter plastic button, a 7-inch stainless steel pin, a 2.5-inch diameter plastic washer, and a cotter hitch pin.

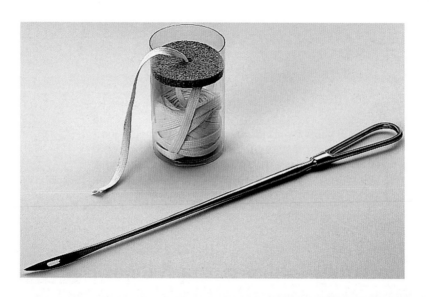

Prolapse Instruments—Umbilical Tape With a Buhner Needle

FUNCTION To suture a large animal vagina closed to prevent a prolapse or to suture the abdomen after surgery.

CHARACTERISTICS Polyester braided "tape" comes in ⅛-, ⅜-, and ¼-inch widths. It is usually packaged in a canister that allows the user to withdraw as much as needed without contaminating the remainder.

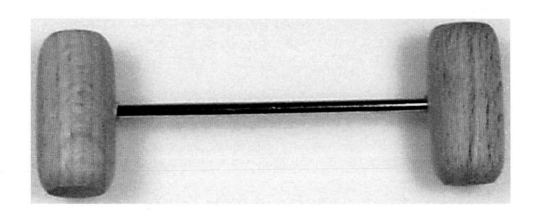

Prolapse Instruments—Vulva Suture Pins

FUNCTION To retain uterine or vaginal prolapse.

CHARACTERISTICS Metal pins are placed across the vulva and stoppered with hard rubber ends that keep the pins in place.

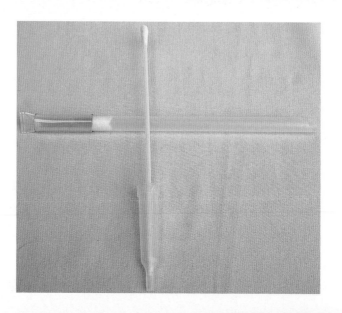

Sample Collection—Culture Swab

FUNCTION To culture the uterus for a variety of screening tests.

CHARACTERISTICS A long plastic tube contains a sterile swab. The tube is inserted into the vagina up to the cervix or even into the uterus. The swab is pushed past a cap or rubber tip that protects it from contamination as it is being inserted. The swab is taken, then pulled back into the protective plastic before being withdrawn.

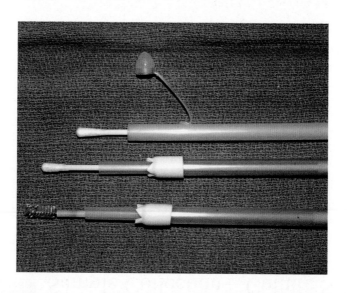

Sample Collection—Uterine Cytology Brush

FUNCTION To gather cells from the cervix.

CHARACTERISTICS Built much like the culture swab, this device has a cytology brush that, when brushed against tissues, collects cells for analysis.

346

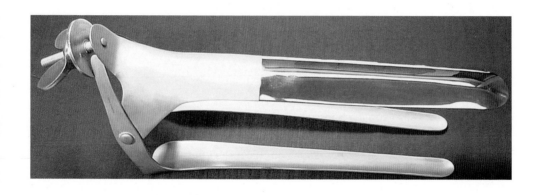

Vaginal Speculum—Polansky

FUNCTION To hold open the labia so the vaginal vault can be viewed, swabs taken, and medication delivered to the uterus. It can also be used during the urinary catheterization of a female.

CHARACTERISTICS The Polansky speculum is opened by squeezing the handles after it is inserted into the vaginal vault. It can be lock open by turning the knob located at the end of the instrument. This speculum can be used on all large animals.

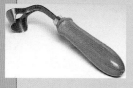

CHAPTER 10

Bovine and Equine Hoof Care Instruments

This chapter covers instruments that are used for cattle and horses to care for their hooves.

Subcategory—General Use of Hoof Instruments

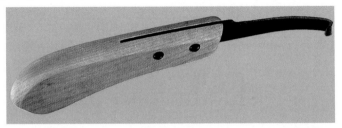

Right handed

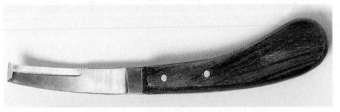

Left handed

Hoof Knife

FUNCTION To trim the frog and sole of an animal's foot.

CHARACTERISTICS A sharp blade on a wooden handle is used to trim away the excess frog and sole after the hoof is shaped. Right- and left-handed blades are available.

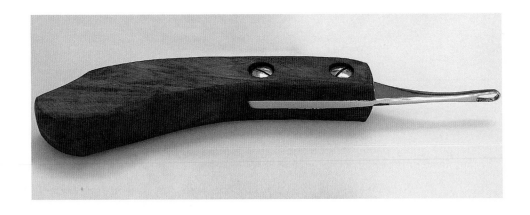

Hoof Abscess Knife

FUNCTION To curette a small hoof abscess.

CHARACTERISTICS A very small, sharp loop is attached to an ergonomic handle; it clears out the area of the abscess.

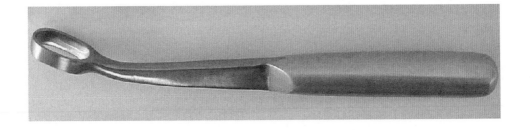

Hoof Groover

FUNCTION To curette a hoof abscess.

CHARACTERISTICS This elliptical, doughnut-shaped blade is attached to a handle and is angled so that it can get into abscessed areas of the hoof.

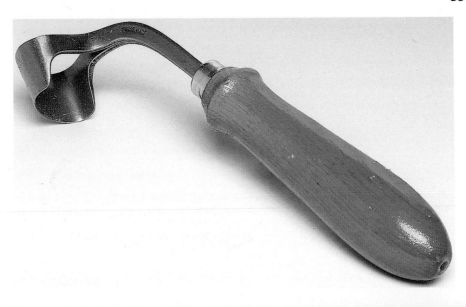

Swiss Hoof Knife

FUNCTION To trim the sole of an animal's foot.

CHARACTERISTICS An oval, sharp blade on a wooden handle is used to trim away the excess sole after the hoof is shaped. A larger version is simply called an oval hoof knife.

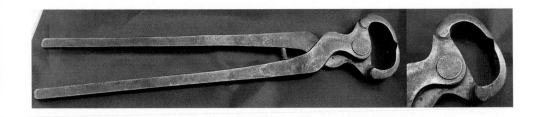

Hoof Nipper

FUNCTION To shape hooves to their normal size in cattle and horses.

COMMON NAME Nippers

CHARACTERISTICS Both jaws are sharp edged, which allows the user to remove fairly large pieces of hoof. The nipper is usually used after the trimmer to form the hoof more closely to the desired shape.

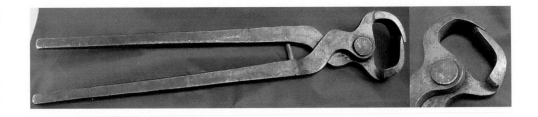

Hoof Parer

FUNCTION To shape a hoof to its normal size in cattle and horses.

COMMON NAME Parer

CHARACTERISTICS One jaw has a sharp edge, the other has a block edge. Working much like a paring knife, this instrument can make small, precise slices off the hoof wall.

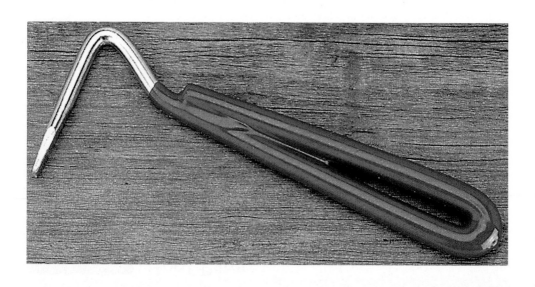

Hoof Pick

FUNCTION To remove debris, mud, and rocks from the hooves before examining them.

CHARACTERISTICS A flat-edged hook has an easy-to-grip handle. The hook part is used to dig and flip debris out of the nooks and crannies of the hoof.

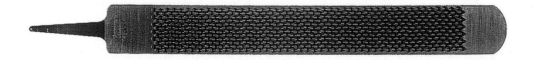

Hoof Rasp

FUNCTION To smooth the rough edges of the hoof wall after trimming.

COMMON NAME Rasp

CHARACTERISTICS A flat piece of heavy metal has two surfaces; one is a rough surface to take down large grooves; the other is a fine surface to put the finishing touches to smooth the hoof wall. The rasp is much like a wood file or a nail file for humans.

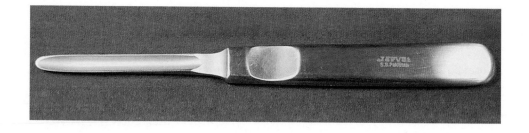

Hoof Searcher

FUNCTION To check for holes or abscesses in the sole of an animal's hoof.

CHARACTERISTICS A straight probe is attached to a handle. The probe is placed into the holes to measure depth and to release the abscess.

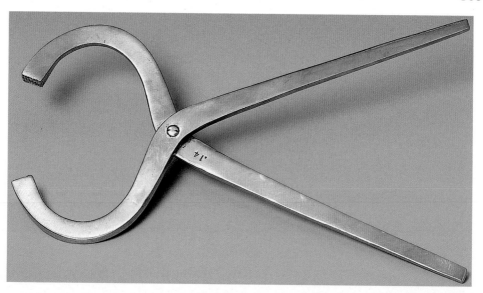

Hoof Tester

FUNCTION To check through a hoof wall for abscesses or sore spots.

CHARACTERISTICS Two jaws are curved so they fit around a hoof; they are attached to handles. The jaws are placed on the hoof wall and sole and squeezed. If the animal reacts, the presence of an abscess is to be suspected.

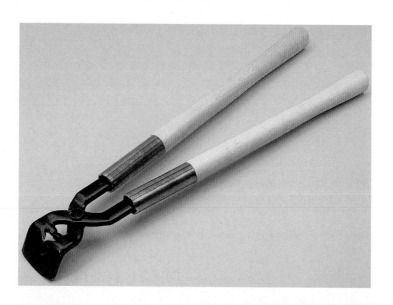

Hoof Trimmers—Long-Handled or Squire Hoof Trimmers

FUNCTION To rough-cut long hooves of cattle and horses while the foot is on the ground.

COMMON NAME Hoof trimmer

CHARACTERISTICS Two sharp blades are placed on 30-inch handles, which allow the user to stand at a distance and use the knees to assist in squeezing the handles together. The trimmer removes large pieces of overgrown hoof so that the smaller trimmers can be utilized to shape the hoof.

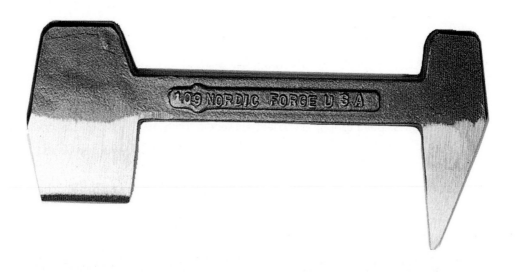

Subcategory—Horse Shoeing and Hoof Therapy Instruments

Clinch cutter

FUNCTION To cut the bent part of a nail that holds the shoe tightly to the foot.

CHARACTERISTICS This instrument has two edges that are sharp enough to cut through the nail that holds the shoe in place. A hammer is used to strike the top of the instrument.

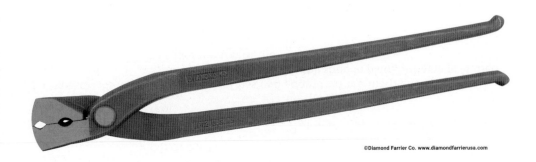

©Diamond Farrier Co. www.diamondfarrierusa.com

Crease Nail Puller

FUNCTION Removes nails from the crease of shoes.

CHARACTERISTICS The jaws are designed to get into the crease of a shoe and pull out the nails holding the shoe to the hoof wall.

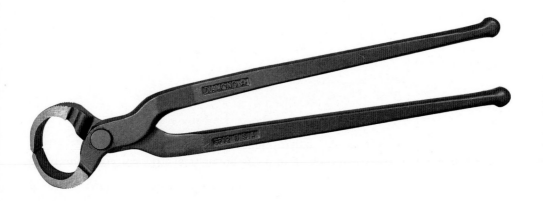

Shoe Puller and Spreader Combination

FUNCTION   Removes shoes from horse hooves.

CHARACTERISTICS   There are sharp teeth on the outside edge for ease in spreading most shoe sizes and styles. It is also used to cut nails.

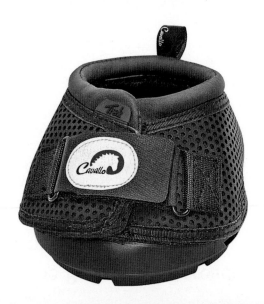

Easy Boot for Horses

FUNCTION   Protect a hoof if injured or to use as a temporary shoe.

CHARACTERISTIC   A rubber boot that fits over a horse's entire hoof. Careful measurements must be taken to get the correct size for each individual horse.

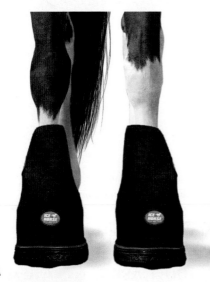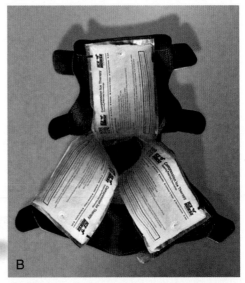

A

B

Hoof Ice Boot—Horse Therapy Boot

FUNCTION Ice or protect hooves that have been injured or strained.

CHARACTERISTICS (A) shows the boot on the horse's foot. The boot wraps around the hoof providing protection or icing from the coronary band to the toe. (B) shows the interior of the boot with the ice bags in place. The ice packs are reusable, and the nonslip rubber sole can be used with a wound pad or wedge.

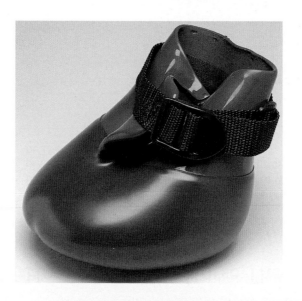

Subcategory—Hoof Instruments for Cattle

Cow boot

FUNCTION To protect a foot that has lost part or all of a hoof.

CHARACTERISTICS This rubber boot is designed to fit over an animal's foot and be laced up, much like a human's overshoe.

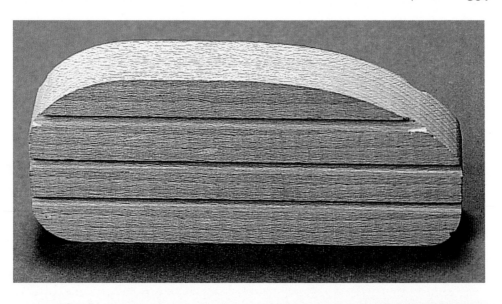

Hoof Blocks

FUNCTION To help a cow that has injured a hoof by protecting the injured hoof.

CHARACTERISTICS Hoof blocks are applied to the uninjured claw to take the weight off the injured claw. They are adhered to the hoof by a special acrylic that can also be used to fix a quarter crack or other hoof abnormality in a horse.

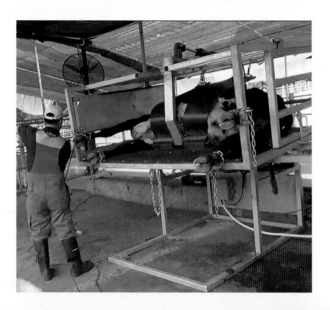

Hoof-Trimming Table

FUNCTION To put a cow into lateral recumbency so as to facilitate access to the hooves for trimming or treatment.

CHARACTERISTICS The table stands upright; the animal is placed alongside the tabletop and strapped into place. The table is then moved into a horizontal position. The animal is often sedated to keep it from struggling.

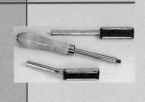

CHAPTER 11

Instruments Used on Equines

This chapter covers instruments used to restrain, treat, and care for horses.

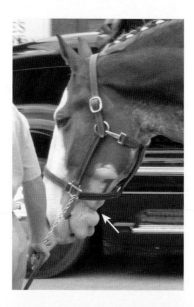

INSTRUMENT # Chain Shank

FUNCTION To provide greater control over a horse by the application of mild pain.

CHARACTERISTICS A flat chain is attached to a clip at one end and to a leather, nylon, or rope lead on the other. (The arrow is pointing at the chain shank under the chin.) The clip end is brought through the side ring on the left side of the halter and over the nose and is clipped to the opposite side ring. A sharp tug on the lead makes the chain dig into the horse's nose. It should be used carefully and with much thought. It can also be used on halters for show cattle (as pictured).

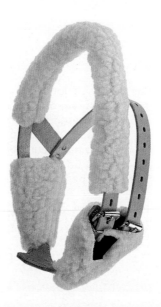

Cribbing Strap

FUNCTION   To prevent a horse from cribbing. Cribbing is when a horse sets its incisors on a fence rail and sucks in air. This is a vice that can affect the horse's endurance.

CHARACTERISTICS   A series of straps is designed to fit around a horse's neck and chin. A strap applies pressure to the larynx only when the horse attempts to crib.

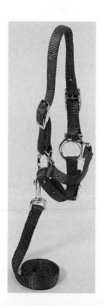

Halter

FUNCTION To provide a means of controlling the horse's head while performing various procedures.

CHARACTERISTICS A series of leather, nylon, or rope straps is designed to go over the nose and around the neck. The halter must be fitted to the horse so that the noseband is below the cheekbones but not lower than the end of the nasal bone. The neck strap, which is placed behind the ears, should be tight but not so constrictive that it chokes the horse. It is important to be sure that the center ring, where the lead rope is attached, is centered under the horse's chin.

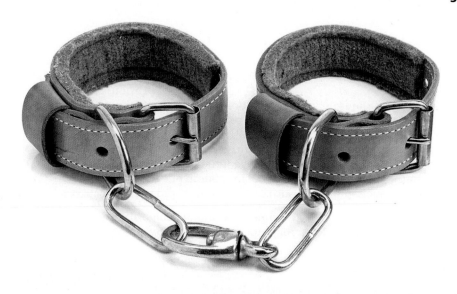

396

Hobbles

FUNCTION To prevent a horse from wandering far away.

CHARACTERISTICS Nylon or leather straps are buckled onto the front legs of the horse. They allow the horse to move but not very fast or very far. It is important to make sure that the legs are square to the body so that the horse does not fall over. Hobbles can also be used on cattle.

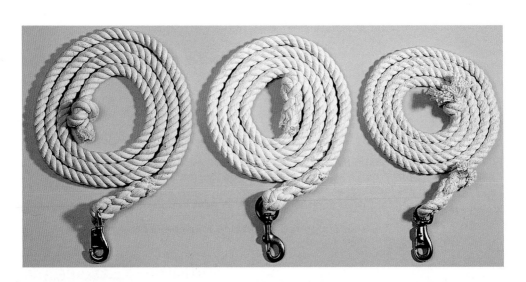

Lead Rope

FUNCTION To lead or tie a horse.

CHARACTERISTICS A leather, nylon, or rope lead that is at least 6 feet in length and has a clip at one end that is used to attach the lead to the center ring on the halter.

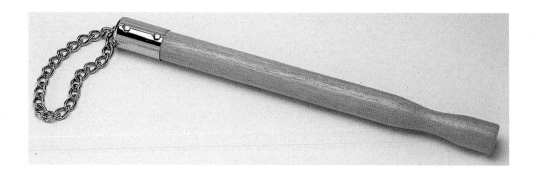

Twitch—Chain

FUNCTION To distract a horse's attention from minor procedures by inflicting mild pain.

CHARACTERISTICS A flat-chain loop is attached to a wooden handle. The upper lip is rolled and pulled through the loop, and the handle is twisted to tighten the chain around the lips. The handle can be rocked or loosened and tightened to add to the distraction. The maximal time during which this instrument is effective is 20 to 30 minutes. This instrument can be equipped with a rope instead of a chain.

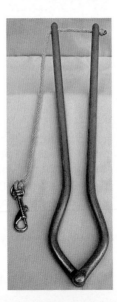

Twitch—Humane

FUNCTION To distract a horse's attention from minor procedures by inflicting mild pain.

CHARACTERISTICS Two aluminum shafts are hinged together; at the hinge is a bow that accommodates the upper lip of a horse. The upper lip is rolled and pulled through the bow; the handles are brought together and either held or clipped to the halter. The maximal time during which this instrument is effective is 20 to 30 minutes.

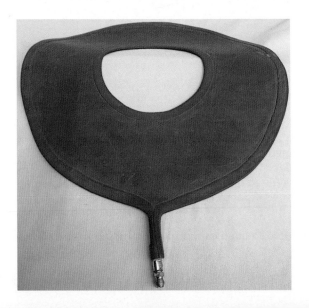

INSTRUMENT Invalid Ring

FUNCTION To cushion a horse's head during surgery. The ring can also be used to cushion the joints of the legs of horses, cattle, and large dogs.

CHARACTERISTICS A red rubber, inner tube–like ring that, when inflated, can be positioned so that the eye or joint is in the center of the hole and the rest of the head or leg is cushioned.

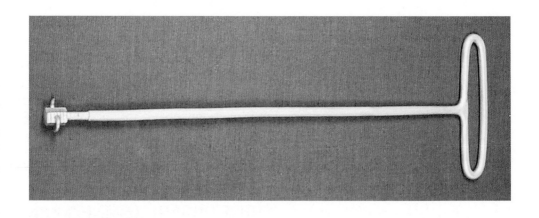

Roaring Burr

FUNCTION To treat equine laryngeal hemiplegia (roaring).

CHARACTERISTICS A rough-surfaced knob is on the end of a shaft that has a T-shaped handle.

Meister, McCullum, Heiner-Rusher, Equivet

Schoupe and Meier wedge speculum

Speculum—Equine Mouth

FUNCTION To hold the mouth open during dental examination and treatment.

CHARACTERISTICS Meister, McCullum, or Heiner-Rusher, or the Equivet mouth wedge; these are metal cups that fit over the incisors and are hinged together. A ratchet device allows the mouth to be pushed open and held open. The entire apparatus is held in place by a noseband and neck strap, unlike a halter. There are a variety of other speculums that fit on one side of the jaw at a time; two of these are the Schoupe equine speculum and the Meier dental wedge.

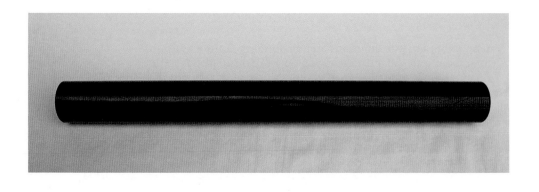

Speculum—Vaginal—Mare

FUNCTION To open the vaginal vault so as to pass swabs or tubes into the uterus or bladder.

CHARACTERISTICS A solid plastic tube that can be sterilized.

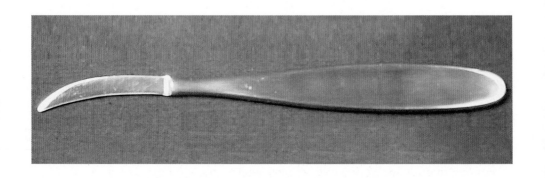

Tenotome Knife

FUNCTION To perform a tenotomy.

CHARACTERISTICS A stainless-steel blade is affixed to a stainless-steel handle. The blade has a blunt or sharp point. The knife can be used without making a surgical incision.

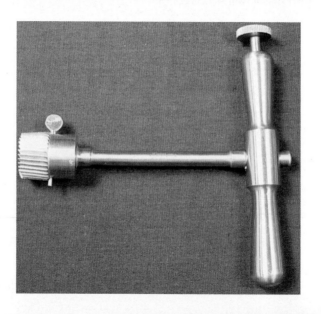

Trephine (Horsley's)

FUNCTION   To drill holes in the cranium or sinus cavities.

CHARACTERISTICS   Sharp-angled blades are arranged in a circle on the end of a long shaft with a T-shaped handle. The blades come in ½-, ¾-, and 1-inch interior diameters.

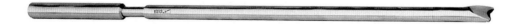

INSTRUMENT **Dental Chisel**

FUNCTION To remove premolar and lower rear molar hooks.

CHARACTERISTICS One end has a notched V that fits around the hook. The other end has a sliding bar or percussion handle that gives extra power to the strike.

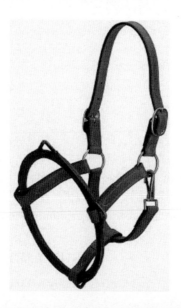

Equine Dental Halter

FUNCTION To provide added restraint during a dental procedure.

CHARACTERISTICS The configuration of this halter is identical to that of a fabric halter except that the noseband is metal rather than nylon. The metal is rounded and covered by leather. Metal loops at the top and bottom of the ring allow the horse's head to be tied for additional restraint or rotation.

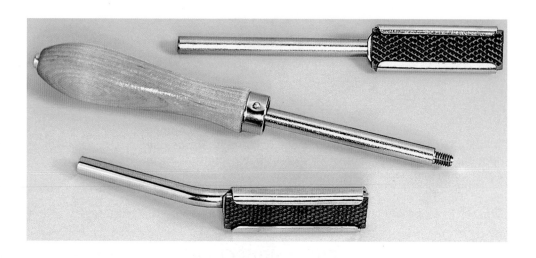

Dental Float

FUNCTION　To smoothen teeth that have rough edges or are overgrown.

COMMON NAME　Floats, tooth floater

CHARACTERISTICS　Float blades are rectangular pieces of metal that are affixed to a straight or angled handle. The blades have rough surfaces in fine, medium, or coarse grains. They can be made of carbide or of tungsten carbide chips. The angled handles facilitate reaching the various sides of a tooth. Many models can be affixed to an electric drill body, which makes the work of floating teeth easier.

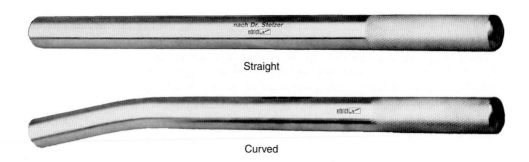

Straight

Curved

Dental Tooth Punch

FUNCTION To remove cheek teeth.

CHARACTERISTICS A hole, drilled with a trephine into the sinus cavity allows the shaft of this instrument to be inserted over the tooth so it can be struck out.

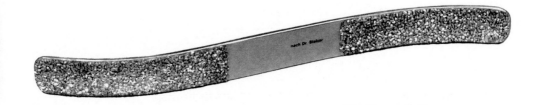

nach Dr. Stelzer

INSTRUMENT Dental Rasp

FUNCTION To give the edges a finished surface.

CHARACTERISTICS Tungsten carbide is found on both ends of this slightly curved and slightly bent instrument. The curves fit the contours of the tooth's surface; the bend allows the rasp to be used on upper and lower teeth.

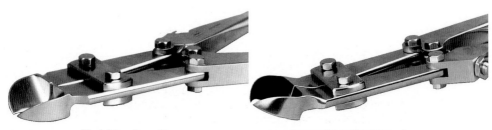

Straight molar cutter

Curved molar cutter

Equine Molar Cutter

FUNCTION To cut or trim molars.

CHARACTERISTICS Heavy straight or angled jaws are situated on handles that allow the user to reach the very back molar.

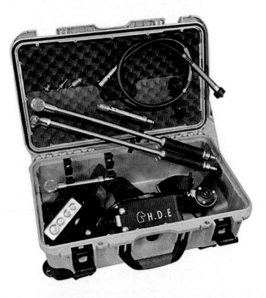

Power Kit—HDE Evolution Power
Kit—Set 4

FUNCTION To perform dental prophylaxis, performance, corrective and surgical equine dentistry.

CHARACTERISTICS This kit comes with a reinforced drive shaft, classic or compact hand pieces, and five attachments to accommodate multiple burrs. This ergonomically comfortable, automated machine allows the veterinary equine dentist to efficiently make corrections to equine teeth.

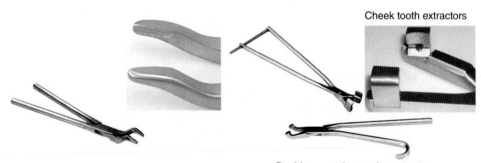

Cheek tooth extractors

Deciduous and premolar extractor

Tooth Extractors

FUNCTION To remove teeth.

CHARACTERISTICS Curved universal small tooth-extracting forceps resemble a pair of needle-nose pliers.

CHARACTERISTICS A cheek tooth extractor has a wider jaw to grip more tooth area and a ratchet to hold the instrument tightly to the tooth. One jaw of the forceps swivels, allowing a number of configurations so that the user can choose the one that fits the tooth that must be extracted. The deciduous premolar-extraction forceps have blocky jaws that enable the user to maintain a good grip.

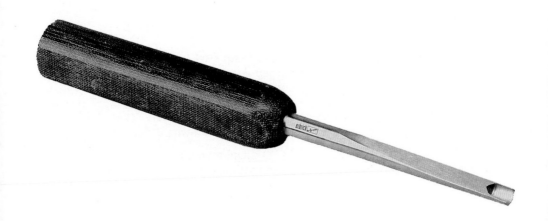

Wolf Tooth Elevator

FUNCTION   To loosen the ligament attachment of a tooth.

CHARACTERISTICS   A tapered shaft is affixed to a handle that can withstand a strike with a mallet. The shaft is designed to slide along the surface of the tooth into the gum tissue.

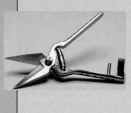

CHAPTER 12

Instruments Used for Pigs, Sheep, and Goats

These instruments are used to restrain, treat, and care for this group of animals.

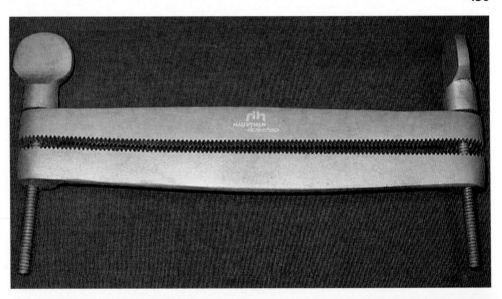

Pig Instruments

Hernia clamp

FUNCTION To retain an umbilical hernia.

CHARACTERISTICS Once the hernia has been reduced, the clamp is applied and allowed to remain in place until the opening has closed and healed.

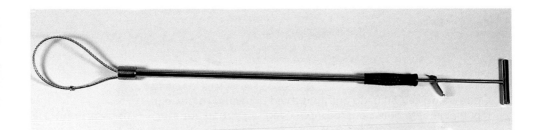

Hog Snare

FUNCTION To capture and hold a hog for venipuncture, injections, or other procedures.

CHARACTERISTICS A looped cable protrudes from one end of this instrument; the other end has a handle that allows the user to tighten the loop once it is placed around the hog's upper jaw. The handler then pulls or leans back, keeping the snare taut; the pig will resist by leaning in the opposite direction. Care must be taken when releasing this instrument to ensure that it does not catch on the canine teeth.

NOTE
Personnel must wear ear protection when using the hog snare because the pigs vocalize at decibels loud enough to cause hearing loss.

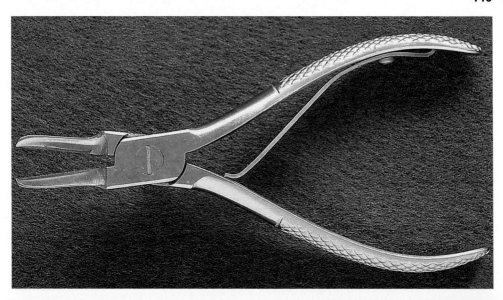

Pig Tooth Nipper

FUNCTION To clip the wolf teeth of piglets.

CHARACTERISTICS Looking much like the side cutters found in most toolboxes, this sharp-jawed instrument allows the user to nip off the teeth that can cause great harm to a sow's udder.

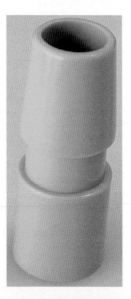

Rectal Prolapse Rings

FUNCTION To retain rectal prolapses.

CHARACTERISTICS These acrylic plastic rings come in a variety of sizes to fit the diameter of the rectum. Ring diameters are 1/2, 5/8, 3/4, 7/8, and 1 inch, all of these are 2 inches long; there is also a ring that is 1¼ inches in diameter and 3 inches long.

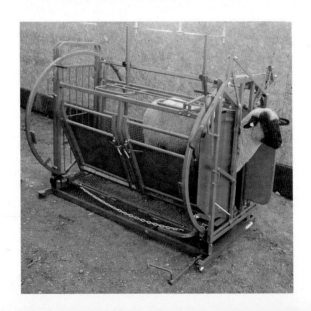

INSTRUMENT # Chute—Deluxe Spin Doctor

FUNCTION To capture, hold, and treat sheep and goats of all sizes.

CHARACTERISTICS This chute has a front and back stop gate, a swing-away false floor, side access panels, and width adjustments to secure any sized sheep or goat. It also rolls to the side for easy access to feet.

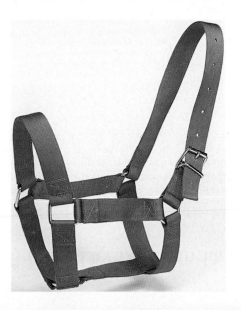

Fabric Show Halter for Sheep

FUNCTION To maintain control of a sheep's head while showing or leading the sheep.

CHARACTERISTICS A headstall with either a chain shank or a cloth nose strap is attached to the sheep's head. The shank or nose strap helps to keep the animal under control.

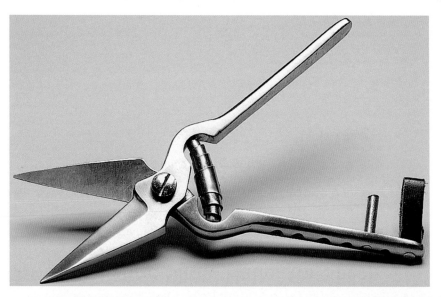

Hoof Trimmer for Sheep and Goats

FUNCTION To trim excess hoof material.

CHARACTERISTICS These shears have long blades that can easily trim one entire side of a hoof at a time. They are available with angled or straight blades that can be replaced.

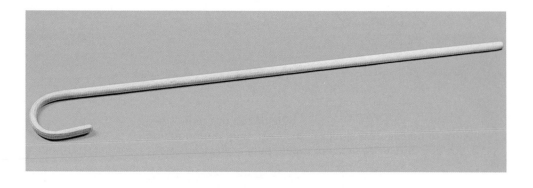

Sheep or Shepherd's Crook

FUNCTION To separate and capture sheep.

CHARACTERISTICS A 60-inch-long rounded staff has a large crook at one end; it is used to snag a back leg or neck to allow the handler to capture a particular sheep.

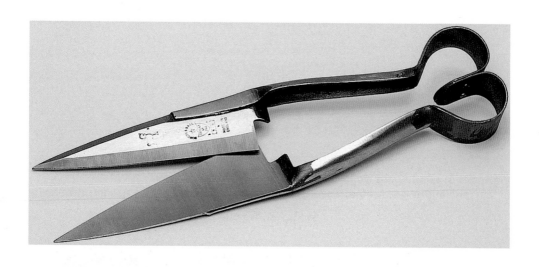

Trimming Shears

FUNCTION   To finish the trimming of sheep.

COMMON NAME   Sheep shears

CHARACTERISTICS   These long shears are used to put finishing touches on the coat for shows and to quickly trim wool from a wound to facilitate care.

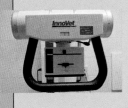

CHAPTER 13

Diagnostic Imaging Instruments and Equipment

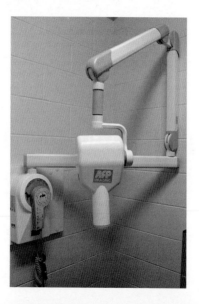

INSTRUMENT Radiography Machine—Dental Stationary

FUNCTION Produces x-rays to penetrate body structures and in turn creates an image of those structures on film or screens.

CHARACTERISTICS This radiography machine focuses the x-ray beam to a very narrow range. It is designed to produce digital radiographs of dental structures.

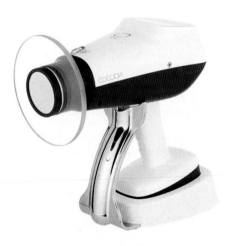

Radiography Machine—Handheld (Dental)

FUNCTION This radiography machine is geared to take dental radiographs but can also be utilized on extremities and limbs. It can be used with film, sensors, or phosphor plates.

CHARACTERISTICS Compact and lightweight, it can be used and stored in a cabinet or drawer. It does not require installation and is cordless. Long battery life allows for hundreds of images from one charge.

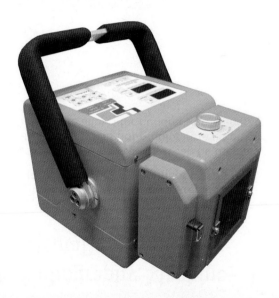

Radiography Machine—Portable

FUNCTION Produces x-rays to penetrate body structures and, in turn, creates an image of those structures on film or screens.

CHARACTERISTICS Same as a stationary radiography machine, except it is designed to be portable for taking radiographs in the field. The tube and console are all in one easily transportable box.

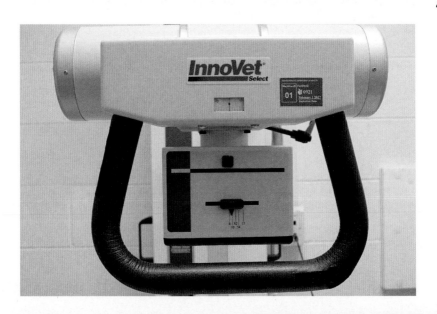

Radiography Machine—Stationary

FUNCTION Produces x-rays to penetrate body structures and, in turn, creates an image of those structures on film or screens.

CHARACTERISTICS The x-rays are produced by a cathode and anode housed within a vacuum tube that is in turn housed in a height-adjustable case. Specific adjustments for kilovolts, amperage, and time are made on a console. The x-rays are focused onto a photographic film that is placed under the area of concern. The film is then processed to reveal the image produced by the x-rays.

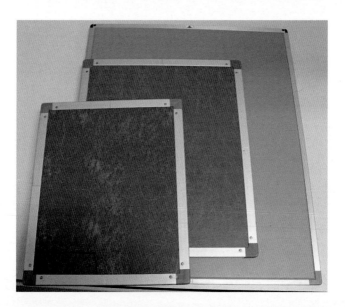

INSTRUMENT

Radiography Cassettes—Film

FUNCTION Film cassettes protect the film from light exposure and damage by the patient. The film is coated with silver bromide or silver idobromide. Computed radiograph (CR) phosphor plates store the image as an electronic charge. Digital radiograph (DR) panels are incorporated into the radiography machine or sensor.

CHARACTERISTICS Film—The x-rays move through the body parts, leaving an impression of the body part on the film. This is done by the conversion of x-rays into light by the intensifying screens inside the cassette. The film then needs to be developed and fixed to see the image and preserve the radiograph. New film is replaced inside the cassettes, taking care not to expose it to regular light, static electricity, bends, or water.

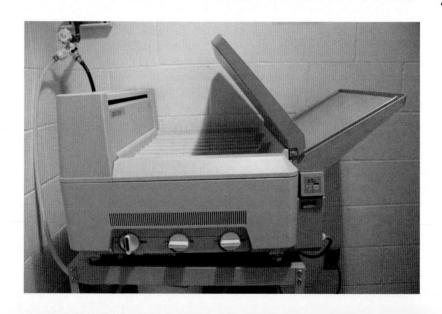

INSTRUMENT Film Processor

FUNCTION Develops film radiographs after they have been exposed to x-rays.

CHARACTERISTICS The film is taken out of the cassette in a dark room and run through a series of developer, fixer, and rinse water tanks. This process takes approximately 2 minutes to produce a wet but visible radiograph.

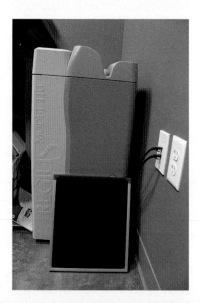

Digital Computed Radiography

FUNCTION The flexible, thin phosphor storage plates are utilized like a traditional film cassette. They are coated with photostimulable compounds that, once exposed to x-rays, trap the image in this compound. To obtain the image, the plate is placed into a reader and scanned by a laser beam and then rendered into a digital image by the computer.

CHARACTERISTICS The plates and readers are usually compatible with existing radiography machines. The plates are available in multiple sizes, making it very flexible for all species. Plate readers are attached to a computer monitor and images are available in about one minute. The plates also need time to clear themselves of residual images and cannot be used immediately to take another x-ray. They can also pick up scatter radiation or background radiation, which can affect the quality of the images, if not cleared and stored properly.

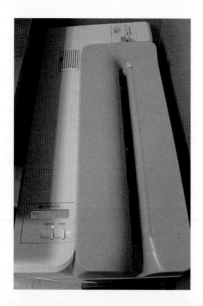

Digital Radiography—Flat Panel

FUNCTION X-ray-sensitive sensors are built into a flat panel, which converts the radiation into an equivalent electric charge and then into a digital image. The digital image is sent directly to a computer giving the veterinarian an instant image of the animal's body.

CHARACTERISTICS The DR image quality is exceptional as the computerized image can be manipulated to compensate for an underexposed or overexposed radiograph. This reduces patient exposure to potentially harmful radiation. Newer DRs are becoming more portable with the development of wireless DR panels. They are quite expensive compared to a good CR setup.

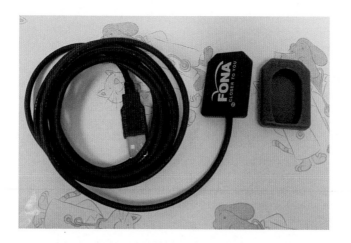

Digital Dental Sensor

FUNCTION Depending on the type of digital sensor, it is attached to the dental radiography unit or directly to the computer, usually with a USB-type cord. Used to obtain dental images.

CHARACTERISTICS The sensor is placed in various positions to obtain different dental views using a digital dental radiography machine.

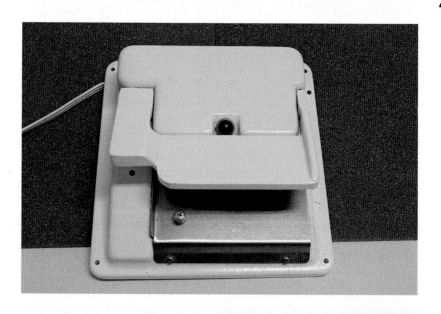

INSTRUMENT **Flasher Labeling Unit**

FUNCTION To identify the patient, owner, clinic, and date on a radiograph.

CHARACTERISTICS A patient identification form is filled out and placed in the flasher; then an exposed film is placed in the flasher and activated. An image of the label is made on the film.

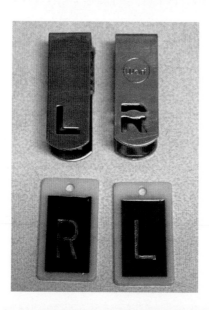

INSTRUMENT   Lead Markers—Directional

FUNCTION   Indicates left and right sides or left and right limbs on a radiograph.

CHARACTERISTICS   Lead letters show up white, as they block the x-rays from penetrating the film or sensor.

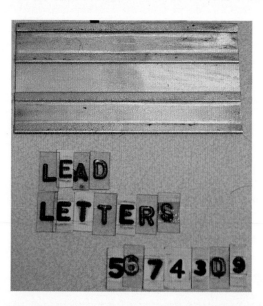

Lead Letters, Numbers, and Holder

FUNCTION To identify the patient, owner, clinic, and date on a radiograph.

CHARACTERISTICS Lead letters and numbers are slid onto the holder and then placed on top of the radiographic cassette. The lead shows up white, as it blocks the x-rays from penetrating the film or sensor.

480

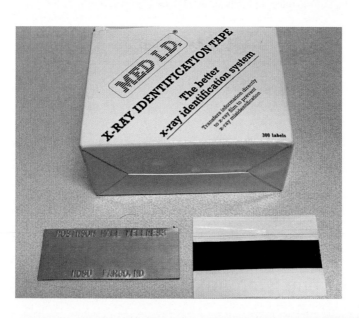

Lead Tape and Holder

FUNCTION To identify the patient, owner, clinic, and date on a radiograph.

CHARACTERISTICS The lead tape is soft, allowing letters to be written onto the tape that will show up white, as they block the x-rays from penetrating the film or sensor.

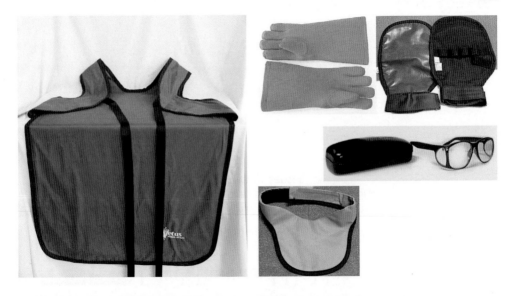

INSTRUMENT

Lead Apron, Gloves, Glasses, and Thyroid Collar

FUNCTION To protect personnel from radiation exposure while they are taking radiographs.

CHARACTERISTICS These pieces of equipment are lined with a thin layer of lead and are worn to protect the body from absorbing radiation. They are considered standard safety equipment.

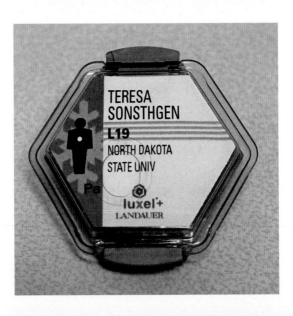

Dosimeters

FUNCTION Record the amount of radiation that personnel are exposed to while taking radiographs.

CHARACTERISTICS The badge is placed at neck or upper chest level outside the protective gear. Most badges are sent in on a monthly basis for processing, and a yearly report of total exposure is sent.

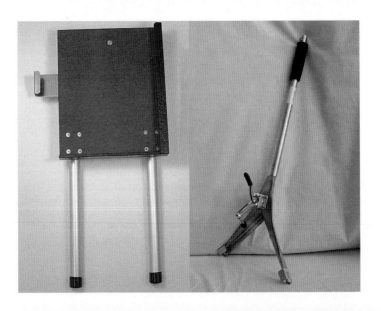

INSTRUMENT **Cassette Holder**

FUNCTION To hold radiographic cassettes at any angle while keeping personnel out of the direct beam.

CHARACTERISTICS A series of clamps is used to hold the film cassette onto a long pole or poles. The cassette can be maneuvered into position behind, to the side of, or between the legs.

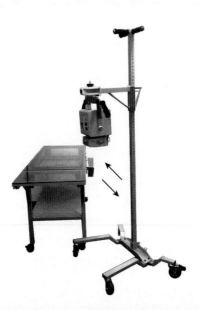

Portable Radiography Machine Stand

FUNCTION Holds and allows for the positioning of a portable radiography machine.

CHARACTERISTICS Usually, a metal stand with adjustable levers allows users to raise and lower a radiography machine and hold it steady to take an x-ray. Often used to assist with radiographs on livestock and horses.

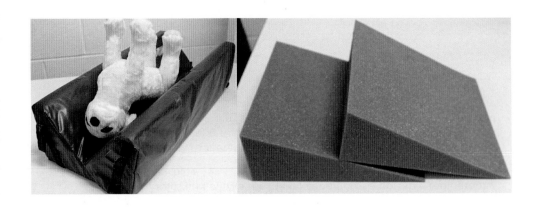

Positioning Devices—General

FUNCTION   Foam padding or troughs that help to position animals correctly for good diagnostic images.

CHARACTERISTICS   The devices can be made of foam with or without a plastic covering for easy cleaning. They may be made of moldable foam, gel, or sand fill to provide hands-free positioning.

492

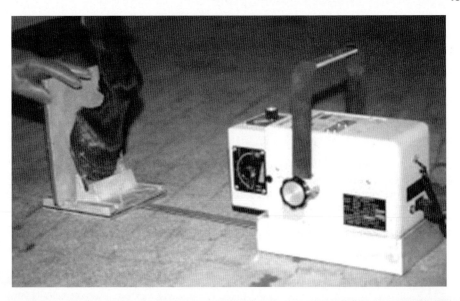

Positioning Devices—Hoof-Angle Gauge

FUNCTION To get an oblique navicular view.

CHARACTERISTICS The stand has a slot into which the toe is placed. It causes the foot to sit at a 45-degree angle. The backstop allows the heel to rest upright, keeping the angle consistent.

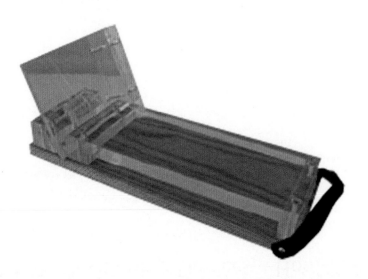

Positioning Devices—Hoof Positioner

FUNCTION To position the hoof for radiographic views of the navicular bone and the third phalanx.

CHARACTERISTICS A heavy-duty plastic platform and an upright brace can be adjusted to facilitate five different views.

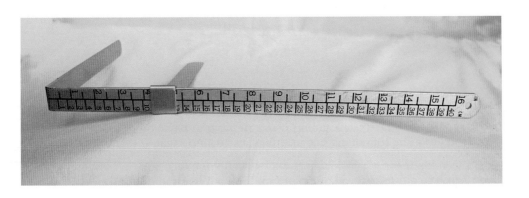

X-Ray Measuring Caliper

FUNCTION To measure an animal's body parts to determine which settings to use on the radiograph machine.

COMMON NAME Caliper

CHARACTERISTICS A sliding T meets the right angle of the caliper. The thickness of the body part is indicated by the graduations on the calipers as shown by the T.

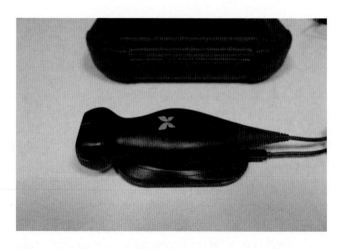

Ultrasound—Wireless and Portable

FUNCTION Performs ultrasounds on all animal species.

CHARACTERISTICS Ultrasounds use high-frequency sound waves to make images of internal body structures, such as fetuses, abdominal organs, muscles, tendons, heart, and blood vessels.

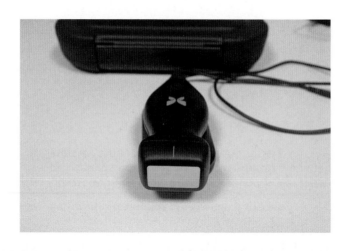

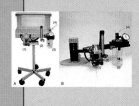

CHAPTER 14

Anesthesiology and Surgical Suite Equipment

This equipment is an essential part of the surgery suite.

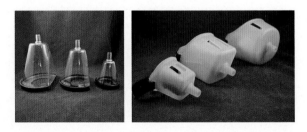

INSTRUMENT **Anesthesia and Oxygen Masks**

FUNCTION To deliver anesthetic gas or oxygen only to an animal that cannot be intubated.

CHARACTERISTICS The mask on the left has a rubber gasket that provides a tight fit over the muzzle. The mask on the right allows for room air to mix with oxygen, which may be a requirement for the animal. This mask is also vented and can be used as a muzzle.

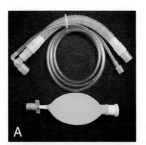

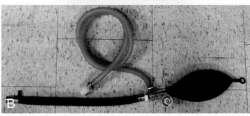

Breathing Circuits—Bain and Ayers—Nonrebreathing

FUNCTION Hoses to connect the patient to a gas anesthesia machine.

CHARACTERISTICS The nonrebreathing circuit allows fresh oxygen and gas anesthesia to be inhaled with every breath. It is used most often for smaller sized patients.

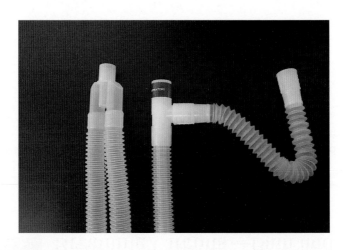

Breathing Circuits—F and Y—Rebreathing

FUNCTION Hoses to connect the animal to a gas anesthesia machine.

CHARACTERISTICS The rebreathing circuit picks up exhaled gases along with fresh oxygen and gas anesthesia with each inhalation.

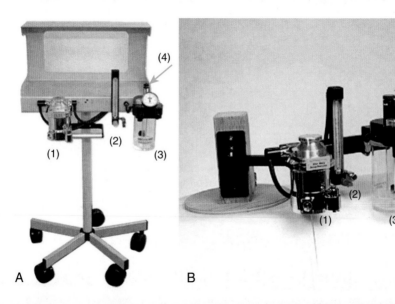

Gas Anesthesia Machine

FUNCTION Equipment used to induce and maintain anesthesia.

CHARACTERISTICS A is an anesthesia machine on a stand for portability and B is a wall-mounted machine. Both have (1) a vaporizer that mixes the anesthetic agent with oxygen and vaporizes it so it can be inhaled, (2) an oxygen flow meter that is set to deliver the appropriate level of oxygen to the patient, (3) a soda lime canister to absorb carbon dioxide from the exhaled breaths, and (4) a pop-off valve and scavenger port to allow excessive gas to be vented and waste gases to be piped from the surgical suite.

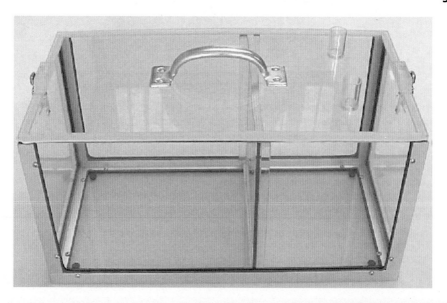

Inhalation Chamber

FUNCTION   To deliver anesthetic gas to an animal too wild or ferocious to handle. It can also be used as a temporary oxygen chamber.

CHARACTERISTICS   A Plexiglas or glass chamber has a lid that allows the attachment of tubes from a gas anesthesia machine. The animal is placed inside, the lid is secured, and the hoses from the gas anesthesia machine are attached. The animal is left in the chamber until unconscious.

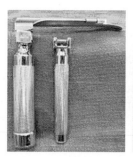
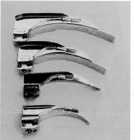
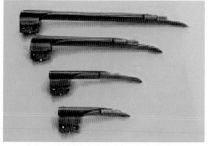

Laryngoscope Handle With Macintosh and Miller Laryngeal Speculums

FUNCTION The handle is used hold laryngeal speculums. The Macintosh laryngeal speculum (B) is used to expose the tracheal opening by applying pressure in front of the epiglottis. The Miller laryngeal speculum (C) is used to expose the tracheal opening by pulling down the epiglottis.

CHARACTERISTICS (A) These handles are designed to hold laryngeal speculums and provide their light source with power. There are two sizes; one requires two C batteries and the other requires two AA batteries.

(B) The Macintosh laryngeal speculum has a curved blade with a flat end. The light source is located midshaft. (C) The Miller laryngeal speculum has a straight blade with a rounded end. The light source is a quarter of the way from the end of the speculum. Both are available in sizes ranging from #0 to #4; #4 has the longest blade.

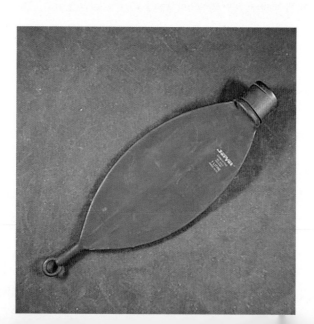

Reservoir Bags

FUNCTION   Used on gas anesthesia machines for manual ventilation and as a visual indicator of breathing by the patient. They also capture exhaled oxygen and gas anesthetic vapors after going through the soda lime cannister.

CHARACTERISTICS   Made of rubber, neoprene or silicon, these bags come in a variety of sizes and are reusable or disposable. They are selected by size according to the weight of the patient. Sizes range from 0.5 to 30 L. The 0.5- to 3-L bags are used on small and exotic animals and the 8- to 30-L bags are used on large and exotic animals.

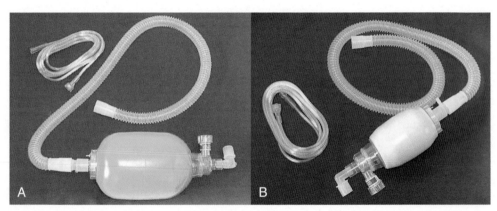

A	B
Large Ambu bag	Small Ambu bag

Resuscitation Bag or Ambu Bag

FUNCTION   To deliver room air or oxygen from a tank to a patient in respiratory distress.

CHARACTERISTICS   Usually used when an endotracheal tube is in place. The large bag is squeezed, forcing room air into the lungs. Bags of various sizes are used according to the size of the patient.

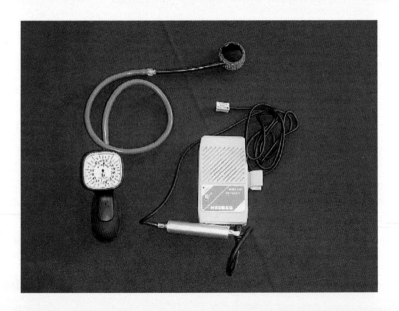

INSTRUMENT Doppler Ultrasonic Blood Flow Monitor

FUNCTION To determine blood pressure.

COMMON NAME Doppler

CHARACTERISTICS The probe is lubricated and secured to shaved skin over an artery. The Doppler picks up the wave ultrasonically as the blood wave passes.

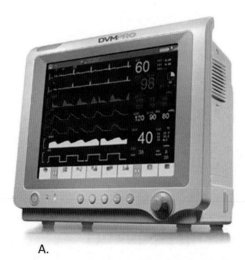

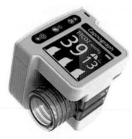

A.

B.

Multiparameter Monitor and
Capnography

FUNCTION An instrument used to gather the vital signs of a patient during
an anesthetic procedure.

CHARACTERISTICS (A) A multiparameter monitor records temperature (T),
pulse (heart rate or pulse rate [PR]), respiration (R), oxygen
saturation, blood pressure (BP and mean atrial pressure), an
electrocardiogram, and end-tidal carbon dioxide. The screen
produces a digital image of each parameter and depending
on the leads used, the multiparameter monitor will produce
reliable results. Each parameter is labeled with the most common
abbreviation. (B) A capnograph measures the concentration or
partial pressure of carbon dioxide.

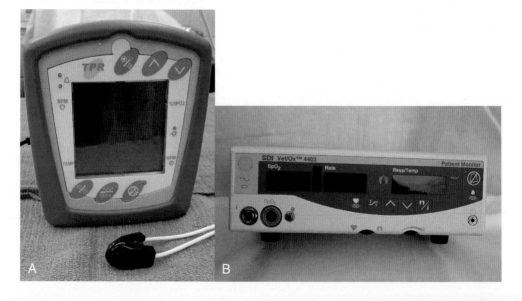

A

B

Pulse Oximeter

FUNCTION   To monitor pulse and respiration rates as well as oxygen saturation and body temperature during surgery.

COMMON NAME   Pulse ox

CHARACTERISTICS   A clamp-like device is attached to the tongue or between the toes of the animal, if the feet are white; it monitors PR and arterial oxygen. Some machines have rectal probes that register the PR; they are useful when dental work is involved. The respiration rate is monitored by a temperature sensor that is placed inside an attachment that connects with the endotracheal tube. As the animal exhales or inhales, the temperature of the air is measured and recorded as a breath. Another attachment to the oximeter records body temperature; a small flexible probe is inserted into the rectum. The oximeter provides an average PR rather than a real-time PR, so checking it manually on occasion is advisable.

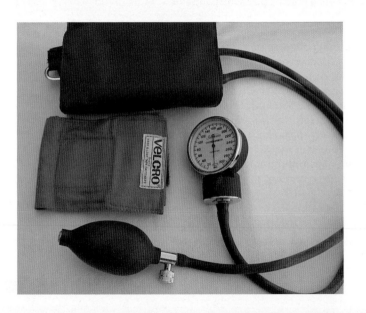

Sphygmomanometer

FUNCTION To determine blood pressure.

COMMON NAME Blood pressure cuff

CHARACTERISTICS A cuff is wrapped around the patient's leg, then inflated by use of the bulb until no sounds can be heard from the dorsal pedal artery. The manometer is slowly released by opening the valve. When the first sound is heard, the number indicated is the systolic pressure. When the sound becomes a pronounced beat, the number indicated is the diastolic pressure. The diastolic number is not as accurate as the systolic number because of the variance in examiners' hearing.

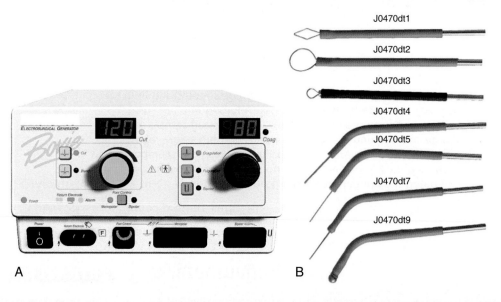

528

J0470dt1

J0470dt2

J0470dt3

J0470dt4

J0470dt5

J0470dt7

J0470dt9

A

B

INSTRUMENT Electrosurgical Generator

FUNCTION To act as part of an electrocautery unit.

CHARACTERISTICS This is one of the many types of electrosurgical units that can be used to cauterize during a surgical procedure and/or to remove surface tumors. There are a variety of tips available for different procedures.

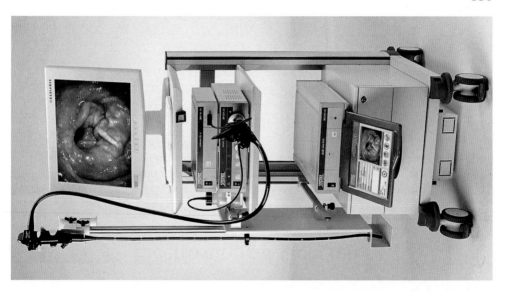

Endoscope

FUNCTION To view the gastrointestinal tract via the oral cavity or rectum or to view the reproductive tract via the vagina. It is also used to perform surgery, biopsy, or culturing through a small incision that allows access to other body cavities.

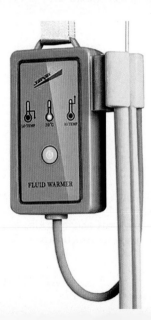

Fluid Warmer

FUNCTION To warm IV fluids before they flow into the patient.

CHARACTERISTICS One of many types of fluid warmers available is shown. The fluid warmer shown is attached to the IV stand, and the IV drip line is placed inside the housing. Some warm the entire bag by being wrapped around it like a "heating pad," or the bag is placed in a warming box.

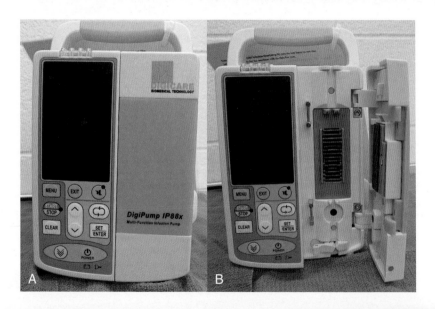

Infusion Pump

FUNCTION To mechanically regulate the flow of fluids into a patient.

CHARACTERISTICS Intravenous tubing is threaded through the machine, which is then programmed to deliver the dose. The user enters the amount of fluid necessary and the time during which it must be delivered. Some models have warmers that keep the fluids above room temperature, a feature that makes their delivery more comfortable for the patient.

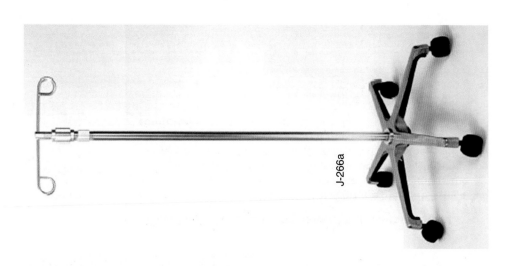

J-266a

Intravenous (IV) Stand

FUNCTION To hold bottles and bags so gravity can deliver the intravenous fluids.

COMMON NAME IV stand

CHARACTERISTICS A stainless-steel stand with two or more hooks that hold bags or bottles of fluid. The shaft of the stand is usually adjustable and the stand usually has wheels.

NOTE
The IV stand can also be used to elevate a limb that needs to be prepped for surgery. A length of rolled gauze is tied to the foot of the affected limb, then elevated and tied to the IV stand. This allows the technician to shave and scrub the entire circumference of the leg and move the patient into surgery

without contaminating the surgical site. The surgeon grasps the leg with a sterile partially unrolled stockinette, the technician cuts the gauze close to the foot, and the surgeon covers the entire foot with the rest of the stockinette.

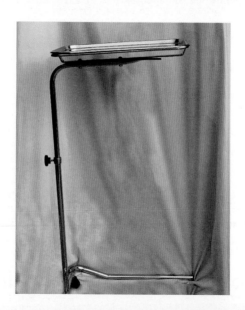

Instrument Stand

FUNCTION To provide a stable surface for the placement of surgical instruments during a procedure.

CHARACTERISTICS This stand has a gooseneck shape so that it can be moved to the surgical table from the end or the sides. Its height is adjustable.

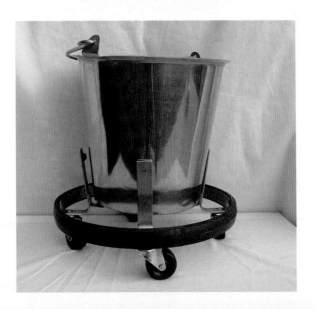

Kick Buckets

FUNCTION To hold garbage generated during surgery.

CHARACTERISTICS Stainless-steel buckets are placed on wheels so a foot can push them easily from one area of the surgery room to another. Because they are stainless steel, they can be disinfected or sterilized easily.

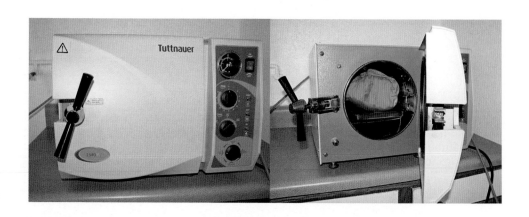

Sterilization—Autoclave

FUNCTION A device used to render objects sterile by steam, heat, and pressure.

CHARACTERISTICS The autoclave consists of (A) a chamber in which specially wrapped objects are placed, (B) a heavy door to seal the chamber, and (C) a water source to create steam. The water source should have distilled water because regular tap water leaves mineral deposits that cause the equipment to fail at some point and the instruments being sterilized become corroded. Each brand of autoclave works a little differently, so it is best to read the owner's manual or get training on the one in your facility before using it.

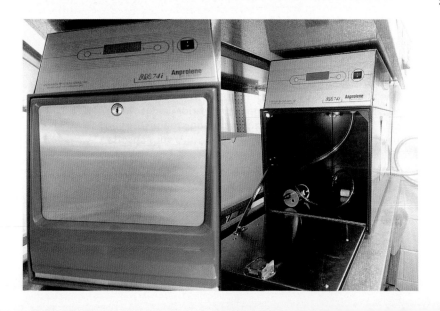

Sterilization—Gas Sterilization Chamber

FUNCTION   A device used to render objects sterile by exposure to chemicals.

CHARACTERISTICS   Ethylene oxide is used to sterilize objects that can be damaged by steam and pressure. It is a highly toxic gas and must be used with extreme caution. Each brand works a little differently, so it is best to read the owner's manual or get training on the one in your facility before using this equipment.

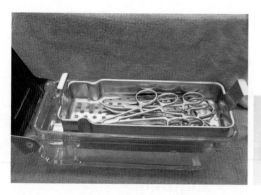

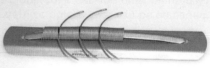

Sterilizer Tray—Bard-Parker With Needle Rack

FUNCTION To hold instruments for cold sterilization. The needle sterilizing racks hold suture needles in an orderly fashion.

CHARACTERISTICS A glass, plastic, or metal tray holds instruments while they are soaking in a cold sterilization solution. Many have a tray that can be lifted and set so that the solution runs off and the surgeon does not touch the solution itself. This prevents accidental contamination of the solution.

The needle sterilizing rack is a spring held in place by a track, which is used as a means of separating suture needles by size and type. The rack is placed in a cold sterilization solution or it can be included in a surgical pack, which ensures that the needles do not inadvertently penetrate the wrapping material.

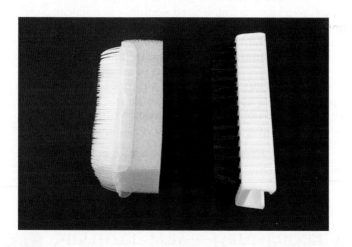

Surgeon's Scrub Brush—Disposable and Reusable

FUNCTION To scrub a surgeon's hands and arms with surgical scrub soap in preparation for surgery.

CHARACTERISTICS The disposable brush has soft bristles and often comes already infused with surgical scrub. The reusable brush has medium to hard bristles on an autoclavable handle. The user needs to pump surgical scrub onto the brush with a foot pump.

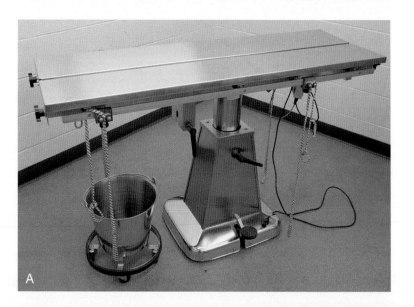

A

Surgical Table

FUNCTION Provides a stable and clean surface to perform surgeries.

CHARACTERISTICS A stainless-steel surgical table can be positioned in a V to keep the patient from rolling from side to side or left flat to accommodate an animal lying on its side. This table has a trough under the center of the table to catch fluids. It has a hook at one end to hold a bucket that can catch fluids, so they do not splatter on the floor. Surgery tables can have either a friction tie-down or a cleat on the four corners that allow ropes attached to the patient to be secured to the table. The table can be raised and lowered by a hydraulic foot pump and tilted in either direction. Some units come with a top that is warmed by an electric unit; if not, they need to be covered to protect the patient from getting cold.

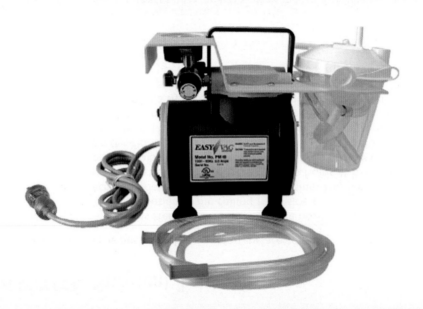

INSTRUMENT	Suction Pump

FUNCTION A device used to remove fluids, tissues, and gases from the surgical patient during surgery.

CHARACTERISTICS This is usually a small motor mounted on a wheeled base with a canister or jar attached to it as a collection device. A small hose with a sterile suction tip is attached to the collection jar. The sterile tip is used to collect fluids and gases during the surgical procedure. After the procedure, it can be used to collect any fluids that may have run into the collect trough or pail under the surgery table.

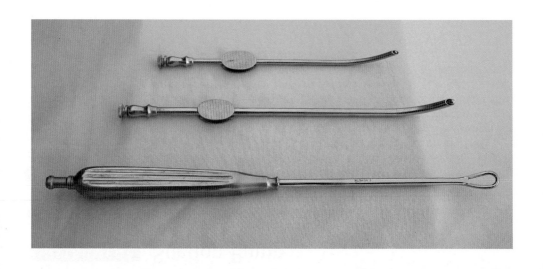

Suction Tips—Yankauer and Frazier

FUNCTION To suction fluids out of surgical fields.

CHARACTERISTICS The Yankauer (bottom instrument) is considered a universal tip. Both suction tips can be attached to a device that suctions the aspirated fluids and carries them to a storage container.

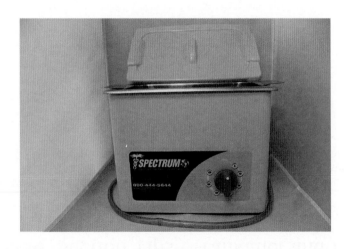

Ultrasonic Cleaner

FUNCTION Cleaning device that generates bubbles that implode on the surface of instruments.

CHARACTERISTICS This device is used to clean microscopic debris from surgical instruments with warm water, a low sudsing detergent, and bubbles created by vibration. The bubbles impode on the surface of the instrument knocking off the debris. This is not a sterilization technique but it does superclean the instruments.

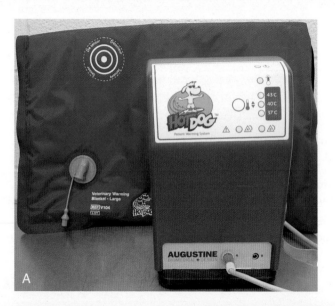

A

Warming Units

FUNCTION Used to maintain or warm a patient's body temperature.

CHARACTERISTICS (A) **Warming Blankets:** The "Hot Dog" patient warming system uses a blanket attached to a generator. The patient is laid directly on the blanket. Another type of blanket system uses a circulating pump, which pumps warm water through a blanket that the patient is laid on. (B) **Convective Warming:** "Equator" and "Bair Hugger" are two brand names of warming devices that blow warm air into a special blanket on which the patient can be laid; the blanket can also be laid over the patient's body. (C) **Towel Warmer:** The "Comfort Zone" towel warmer is a portable device that can warm three to four large towels in about 15 to 20 minutes. These are fine to use; however, the towels tend to cool off quickly.

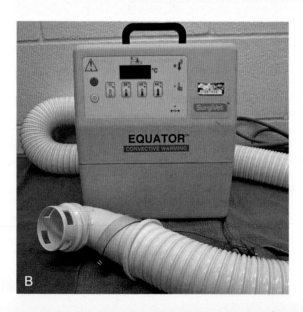

Warming Units (continued)

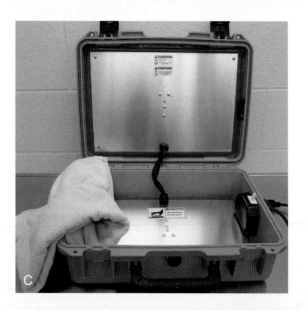

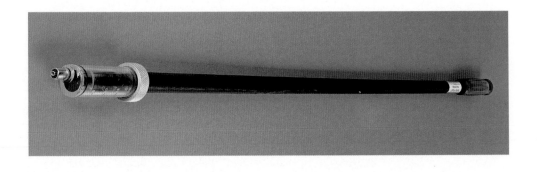

Pole Syringe

FUNCTION To administer a parenteral injection to an animal too wild or ferocious to handle.

CHARACTERISTICS The plunger of a syringe is attached to a long pole. A regular syringe is taken apart and the barrel is attached to the plunger of the pole syringe. The syringe is filled in the normal way, and the handler uses the pole to insert the needle and push the plunger from a safe distance. The plunger section can be changed to accommodate various syringe sizes. These are often used to administer an anesthetic.

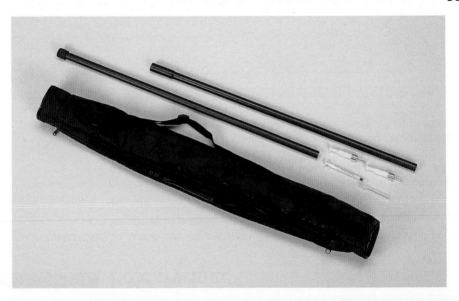

Blow Dart

FUNCTION To propel a dart syringe towards an animal that is too wild or ferocious to handle.

CHARACTERISTICS This hollow tube is designed to accommodate a special syringe that flies by air propulsion and discharges on impact. The tube usually has a mouthpiece on one end. Often used to administer an anesthetic to animals from a safe distance.

PART 2

Surgical Instruments

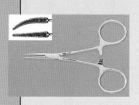

CHAPTER 15

Hemostats and Forceps

Hemostatic forceps, also known as hemostats and clamps, are generally used to grasp blood vessels or to clamp and hold tissues or vessels. The instruments vary in length from 3 to 9 inches and have grooved jaws that give them holding and crushing power. The grooves on most hemostats traverse the length of the jaws; some have grooves running longitudinally, and others have a combination of grooves. Each is equipped with a ratchet or box lock that allows the instrument to be locked and left in place, and all hemostats are available with either straight or curved jaws. Size selection is determined by the size of the blood vessel or tissue bundle to be clamped.

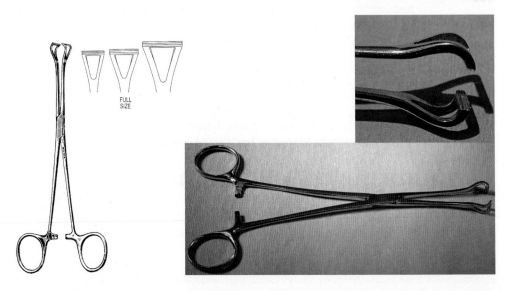

FULL
SIZE

Babcock Intestinal Forceps

FUNCTION To grasp or encircle delicate tissue, such as intestines or uterus, without crushing or traumatizing it.

CHARACTERISTICS Jaws curve out, and grooves run parallel where the jaws meet. These forceps have a lighter jaw compression, which allows atraumatic occlusion. Lengths range from 6¼ to 9½ inches.

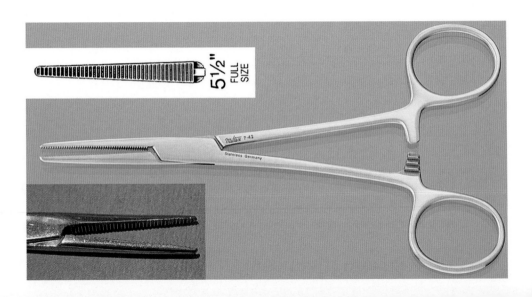

5½"
FULL
SIZE

miltex 7-42

Stainless Germany

Crile Forceps

FUNCTION   To occlude vessels such as small uterine horns or small-to medium-sized blood vessels.

CHARACTERISTICS   A forceps 6½ or 7¼ inches long with transverse grooves on the entire jaw.

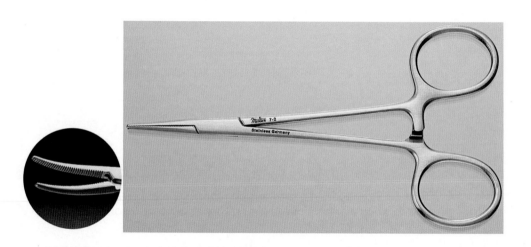

Halsted Mosquito Forceps

FUNCTION To clamp small vessels that must be occluded, crushed, or held firmly in place.

COMMON NAME Mosquito

CHARACTERISTICS A forceps 5½ inches long with transverse grooves on the entire jaw.

NOTE
The most commonly used small hemostat in surgical packs for dogs and cats.

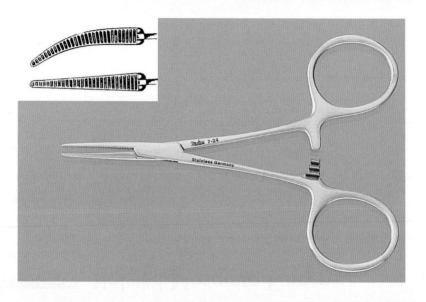

Hartman Mosquito Forceps

FUNCTION   To clamp or occlude small capillaries or vessels that have been cut or are about to be cut.

COMMON NAME   Mosquito

CHARACTERISTICS   A forceps 3½ inches long with transverse grooves on the entire jaw.

NOTE
It is sometimes referred to as a mosquito because it is the smallest hemostat with a box lock.

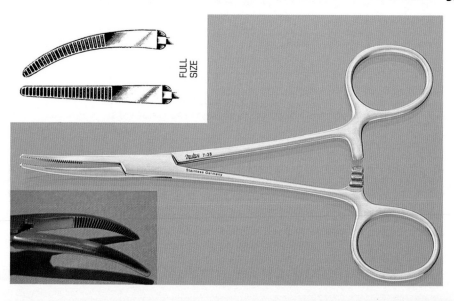

FULL
SIZE

Kelly Forceps

FUNCTION To occlude small-to medium-sized vessels.

CHARACTERISTICS A forceps 6½ inches long with transverse grooves only on the top half of the jaws; the lower half is smooth. The smooth area allows the user to clamp tubing without worrying that the tubing will be cut.

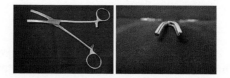

Ferguson Angiotribe Forceps

FUNCTION To powerfully crush and create a fold in the tissues to which it is applied. It is often included in spay packs because it can be applied to uterine horns and spermatic cords.

CHARACTERISTICS One jaw has a raised ridge that runs down the center; the opposite jaw has a groove that accommodates the ridge when the instrument is closed. Both jaws have grooves that provide additional crushing power. The lengths of these forceps are 6½ and 7½ inches.

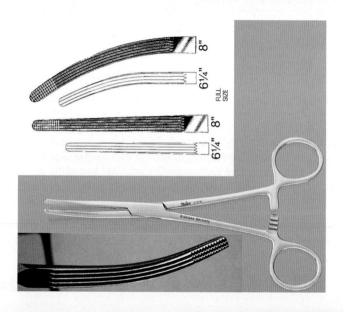

Rochester Carmalt Forceps

FUNCTION   To clamp large tissue bundles that have a lumen or contain blood vessels. When the instrument is placed perpendicular to the blood vessel, it occludes the vessel and prevents blood flow. The other hemostats with transverse grooves can allow blood or body fluids to continue flowing.

COMMON NAME   Rochester

CHARACTERISTICS   The first quarter of the jaws have grooves that run both longitudinal and transverse; the other three-quarters of the jaws have longitudinal grooves only. The tips of the jaws can be used to grasp and crush tissue, whereas the longitudinal grooves allow the user to slip off the hemostat after ligation. For small animals, these forceps are 6¼ to 8 inches long; those used in large animals may be as long as 12 inches.

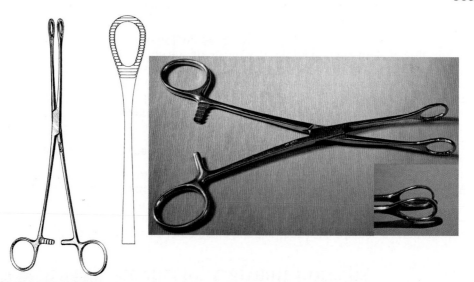

Foerster Sponge-Holding Forceps

FUNCTION To apply the final paint of Betadine solution to a surgical site or to handle sterile dressings to provide hemostasis. Its length allows the user to reach far into a body cavity.

CHARACTERISTICS The oval jaws can be smooth or serrated. The length is usually 7 inches, but they are also available in a 9½-inch length.

NOTE
When using these forceps for hemostasis, it is important to avoid wiping or dragging the gauze across the vessel; doing so can pull the clot away from the vessel and can cause abrasions to the vessel and surrounding tissues.

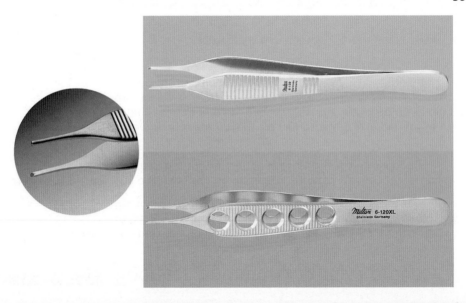

Tissue forceps vary in shape and are classified according to their uses. Most are used to grasp tissue or inanimate objects depending on the type of teeth or jaws they have and whether they have a ratchet or are held closed by the user.

INSTRUMENT

Adson Tissue Forceps

FUNCTION To pick up, hold, and maneuver delicate tissues.

CHARACTERISTICS The very fine teeth on each of the tines cause minimal trauma when a user is picking up and temporarily holding soft tissues. The usual length of the Adson forceps is 4¾ inches; they are available in 1 × 2 and 2 × 3 tooth arrangements, with either standard or delicate tines. They have a wide blade to allow thumb and finger pressure without fear of the tissues rotating out from between the fingers.

592

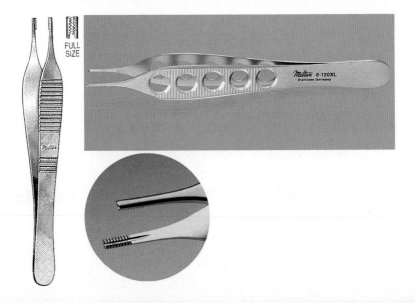

FULL
SIZE

Miltex 6-120XL
Stainless Germany

Brown-Adson Tissue Forceps

FUNCTION To pick up, hold, and maneuver delicate tissues.

CHARACTERISTICS There are two rows of nine teeth on each tine that interlock when closed; each tine is 4¾ inches long with the same handle design as the Adson.

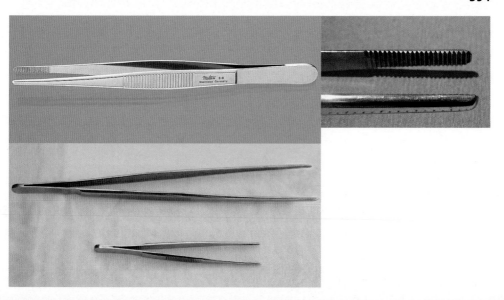

Dressing Forceps

FUNCTION   To grasp inanimate objects such as dressings or nonviable tissues; this type of forceps cause significant damage to viable tissues.

CHARACTERISTICS   The dressing forceps have transverse grooves that run across the tines. These forceps can be ordered with fine or fluted handles and can have extra-narrow tips. Lengths vary from 4½ to 12 inches.

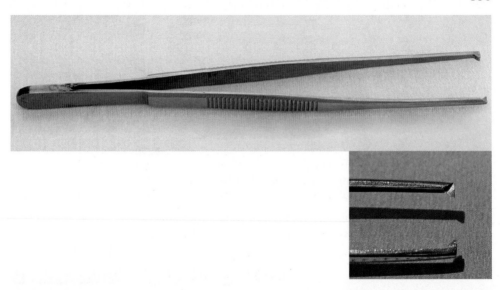

Tissue Forceps—Rat-Tooth

*FUNCTION To grasp skin and other dense tissues to place sutures. Forceps of this description can cause extensive damage to delicate tissues.

CHARACTERISTICS Two tines are connected at one end and are designed to remain open if pressure is not applied by fingers to close the tines. These tines have large teeth; one tooth fits in between two teeth on the opposite tine. The rat-tooth forceps can be ordered with serrated or fluted handles, and the lengths vary from 4½ to 12 inches. Teeth arrangements include 1 × 2, 2 × 3, 3 × 4, and 4 × 5 teeth. These forceps can also be ordered with extra-fine tips.

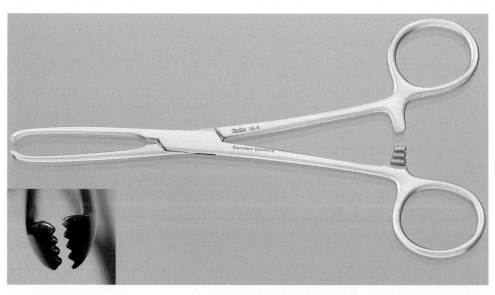

Tissue Forceps—Allis

FUNCTION To hold with maximal power. However, they can cause tissue trauma in the process.

CHARACTERISTICS These forceps have a box lock and jaws with small teeth that are arranged so that the teeth are perpendicular to the pull. It is recommended that viscera not be grasped or held with these forceps because it can result in extensive damage. The length is 6 inches; teeth can be 3×4, 4×5, or 5×6 on each tip.

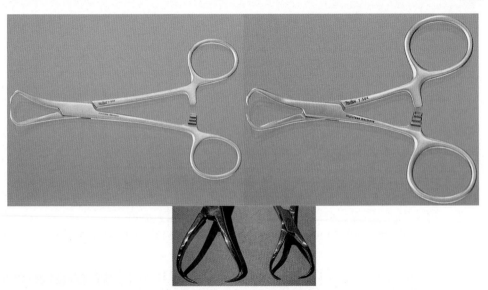

INSTRUMENT Backhaus Towel Forceps

FUNCTION To secure the drapes to a patient's skin by means of a small puncture. These forceps can also be used to grasp tough tissues and reduce small bone fractures.

CHARACTERISTICS Sharply pointed tips curve around and touch each other. They lock into place with a box lock. Lengths include 3½ (right) and 5½ (left) inches. A variation of the same instrument are the Roeder towel forceps, which have a metal bead on each tine. The beads prevent deep punctures to the skin and keep the drape from sliding toward the box lock.

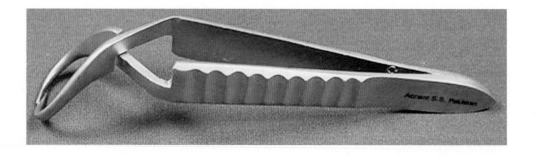

Jones Towel Forceps

FUNCTION To secure drapes to the patient's skin by means of a small puncture.

CHARACTERISTICS Sharply pointed tips curve around and touch each other. The forceps lock into place by means of pressure instead of a box lock and are available in 2½- and 3½-inch lengths.

NOTE
One of the most commonly used large hemostats in surgical packs for dogs and cats.

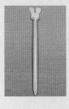

CHAPTER 16

Instruments in Surgical Packs

This chapter covers instruments that are included in most traditional surgical packs but do not fit the criteria necessary to be defined as a hemostat or forceps. It also includes some miscellaneous instruments that may also be included in a surgical pack, depending on the procedure being performed.

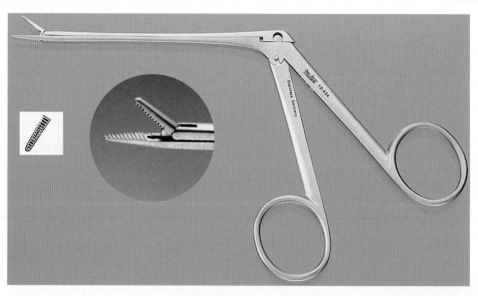

INSTRUMENT Alligator Forceps

FUNCTION To reach deep into an animal's body to retrieve a foreign object.

CHARACTERISTICS This distinctive instrument has a long narrow shaft that ends in tiny grasping jaws. The jaws are opened and closed by handles that resemble forceps. The jaws may be serrated or cross-hatched or may have 1×2 teeth on the very tips. The shafts may be 3½, 5½, 8, or 12 inches long.

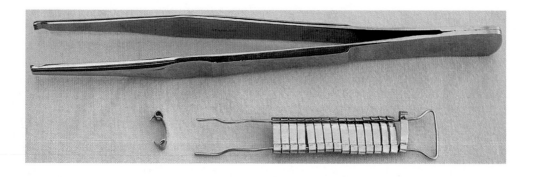

Michel Wound Clip and Applying Forceps

FUNCTION   The clips are used to hold wounds together or to roll out eyelids in cases of entropion.

The forceps are used to apply or remove Michel wound clips.

CHARACTERISTICS   The forceps come in two designs. One looks very much like thumb forceps, except that the tips are cupped to hold the clips. The other has handles with a removing device at one end and the applying cups at the ends of the handles. The forceps are used in closing wounds and are often used for entropion in sheep. The metal clips are small with sharp prongs that fold over incision sites or wound edges to hold them together.

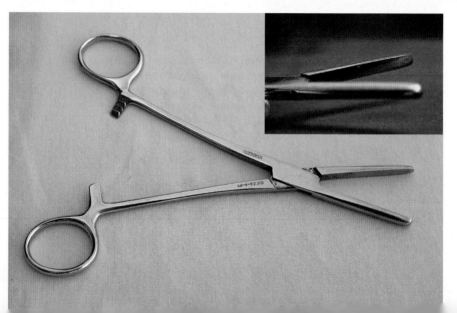

Presbyterian Hospital Occluding Forceps

FUNCTION To clamp rubber tubing without cutting through it.

CHARACTERISTICS The jaws on these forceps are smooth.

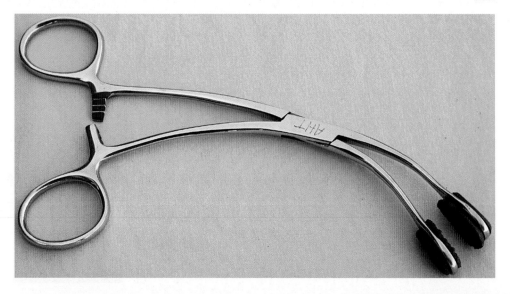

Young Tongue-Seizing Forceps

FUNCTION To grasp and hold the tongue atraumatically.

CHARACTERISTICS Soft rubber inserts on the jaws of these forceps protect the tongue as the instrument's jaws are closed. The instrument is usually curved and approximately 7 inches long. The rubber inserts get hard over time but can be replaced with new ones by simply popping out the old inserts and popping in the new ones.

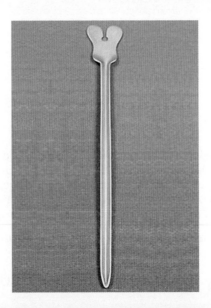

INSTRUMENT Groove Director

FUNCTION To shield underlying tissues while making an incision and to help make a straight incision line. A small stab incision is made through the skin and muscle layer using a scalpel blade. The groove director is introduced into the small incision and held parallel to the muscle layer. The trough is used to guide the scalpel as it makes the incision.

CHARACTERISTICS A heart-shaped handle lies at one end of an open, trough-like, tapered tube that extends along its length.

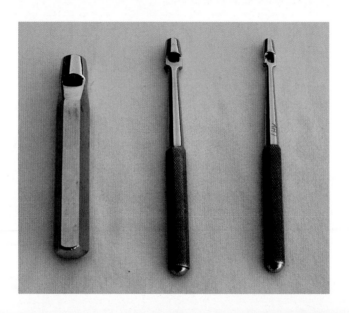

Keyes Dermal Punch

FUNCTION To obtain a dermal biopsy.

COMMON NAME Dermal punch, punch

CHARACTERISTICS Sharp edges have a variety of diameters, including 2, 3, 4, 6, and 8 mm.

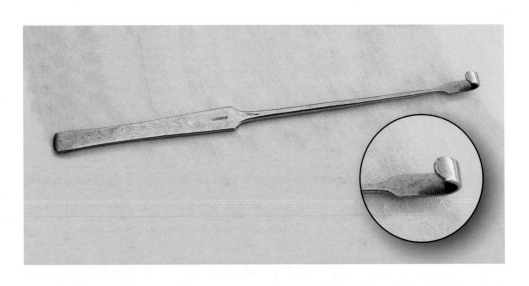

Snook Ovariectomy Hook

FUNCTION To retrieve the uterine horn from within a small animal. This instrument allows the surgeon to make an incision smaller than a finger can fit into.

COMMON NAME Snook hook

CHARACTERISTICS This instrument is 8 inches long and has a flat, rounded hook at the end.

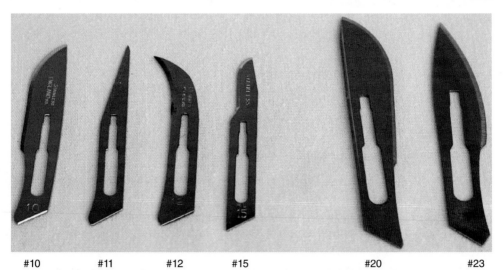

#10   #11   #12   #15   #20   #23

Fit onto a #3 scalpel handle   Fit onto a #4 or #8 scalpel handle

Scalpel Blades—#10, #11, #12, #15, #20, #23

FUNCTION   To make incisions, cut tissues, or debride dead tissue from wounds.

CHARACTERISTICS   Each blade has its own shape and function.

#10—A general blade that is used for most procedures in small animals; fits a #3 handle.

#11—Used to puncture the skin, open an artery, and sever ligaments; fits a #3 handle.

#12—Used to lance an abscess; fits a #3 handle.

#15—Used for small, precise, or curved incisions; commonly used to declaw cats; fits a #3 handle.

#20 and #23—General blades used for most procedures in large animals; fit a #4 or #8 handle.

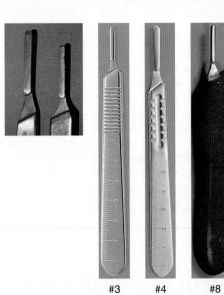

#3 #4 #8

Scalpel Handles—#3, #4, and #8

FUNCTION To incise and transect. These handles hold a variety of sizes of surgical blades firmly in place while allowing the user to maneuver and maintain a comfortable grip. The #3 handle is used primarily for surgery in small animals; the #4 and #8 handles are used for surgery in large animals.

CHARACTERISTICS Handles #3 and #4 are spatula-like and have ribbed grip areas. The #8 handle is made of plastic and contoured to fit the hand, making the user's grip on it more secure in cold temperatures. Each handle size has a blade seat of a different size.

CAUTION
Never use your fingers to place or remove a blade from the handle. Grasp the noncutting edge of the blade with a hemostat or needle holder, and line the slant on the bottom of the blade with the slant on the handle. Then, slide the blade into the grooves on

Scalpel Handles—#3, #4, and #8 (continued)

the tip of the handle until it clicks into the seat. To remove the blade with a hemostat or needle holder, grasp the bottom corner of the blade and lift and slide it off the tip of the handle. Dispose the blade into a sharps container.

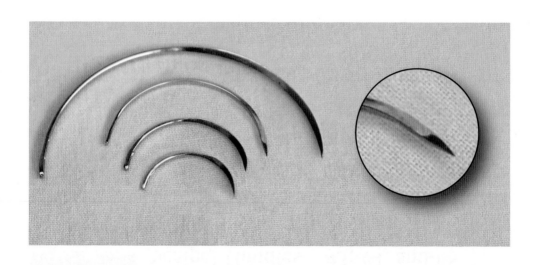

Suture needles are used to introduce suture material into tissues. They come in a variety of sizes, shapes, and thicknesses; a particular needle chosen is determined by the type of tissue to be sutured and the type of suture material to be used.

INSTRUMENT

Half-Circle Cutting-Edge Suture Needle

FUNCTION To suture skin, tendons, and ligaments.

CHARACTERISTICS This needle is triangular and has cutting edges on all three sides or has a flat cutting surface at the tip that gradually forms a triangle as it gets closer to the eye. The needle actually slices a flat line into the tissue as it is passed. This can weaken soft tissue like muscle and allow serum to accumulate on both sides of the tissue. These needles are available in ½- and 3⁄8-inch diameters.

INSTRUMENT **Half-Circle Cutting-Edge Suture Needle (continued)**

Sizes start at 2, the largest, and decrease by increments of 2; size 20 is the smallest needle. There are also cutting-edge suture needles for large animals that are measured in inches, starting at 3 inches and progressing to 6 inches in length.

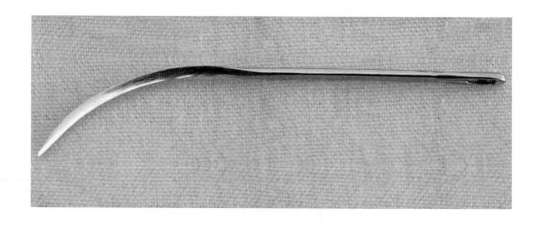

Half-Curved Cutting-Edge Suture Needle

FUNCTION To suture skin, tendons, and ligaments.

CHARACTERISTICS This needle has a straight shaft that ends in a half-curve.

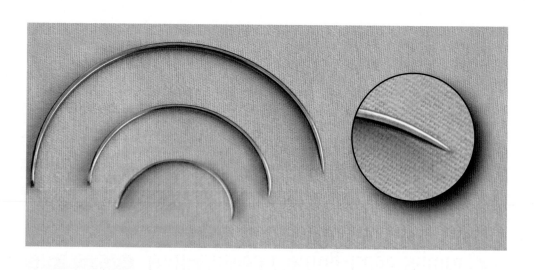

Half-Circle Taper-Point Suture Needle (Ferguson)

FUNCTION To suture organs and vessels.

CHARACTERISTICS This needle is round from point to eye. The rationale is to select suture material of the same size diameter as the needle. When the needle is pushed through the tissue, the suture material fills the resulting hole. This reduces trauma to the tissue and helps prevent leakage, if the organ or vessel happens to have a lumen. These needles are available in ½- and 3⁄8-inch diameters. Sizes start at 2, the largest, and decrease by increments of 2; size 20 is the smallest needle. They can also vary in diameter; intestinal needles are fine, while regular surgeons' needles are quite thick.

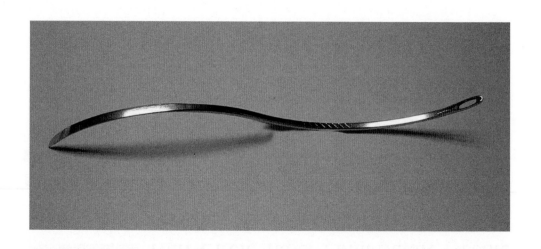

Postmortem Needle

FUNCTION Used to suture the skin on animals that have had a necropsy. Some veterinarians use it to suture large animals' skin after abdominal surgery.

CHARACTERISTICS This large needle has a cutting edge and is curved to allow the veterinarian to grasp it just below the eye and hold it while pushing it through the skin. Large suture material can be used, which can speed up the closure of a necropsied animal or a lengthy incision on a large animal.

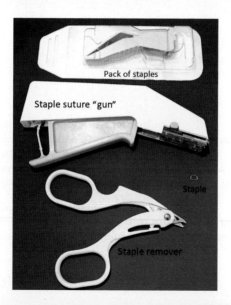

Pack of staples

Staple suture "gun"

Staple

Staple remover

Suture Stapler and Remover

FUNCTION   To close incisions and wound sites with stainless steel staples and remove the staples when the incision or wound has healed.

CHARACTERISTICS   A gun-like instrument is loaded with stainless steel staples, the tips are held against the incision or wound site, and the handles are squeezed to fold a staple over the incision or wound. When the wound has healed, the jaws of the remover are slipped under the staple, the handles are squeezed, and the staple is unfolded and removed from the skin.

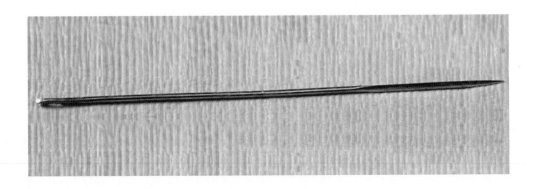

Keith Abdominal Suture Needle

FUNCTION Cutting-edge needles are used to suture skin, tendons, and ligaments.

CHARACTERISTICS This needle is straight.

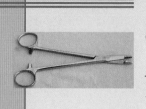

CHAPTER 17

Needle Holders and Scissors

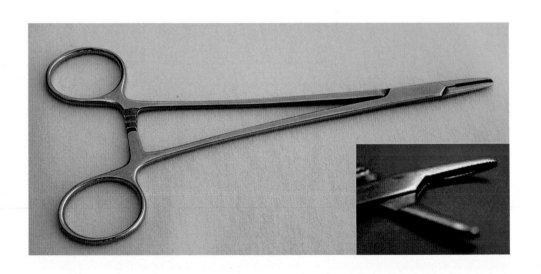

Mayo-Hegar Needle Holder

FUNCTION To drive suture needles through tissue that requires suturing and to assist in tying sutures.

COMMON NAME Needle holder

CHARACTERISTICS Short jaws have grooves that are cross-hatched on the surface, and some models have a longitudinal groove down the centers of the jaws. Cross-hatching provides superior holding power, so the needle does not turn in the jaws. The needle holder has a box lock and may have carbide inserts in the jaws. The inserts can be replaced, if the jaws lose their gripping power; thus extending the life of the needle holder. Needle holders with carbide jaws have gold handles. Lengths include 5¼, 6, 7, 8, 10½, and 12 inches. The size of the needle holder is determined by the size of the needle used. A needle that is too large for a particular needle holder can damage the jaws and the box lock.

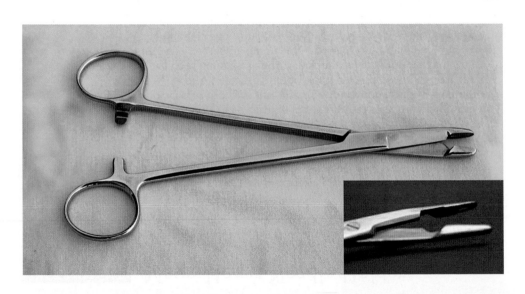

Olson-Hegar Needle Holder—
Scissors Combination

FUNCTION To drive suture needles through tissue that requires suturing and to assist in tying sutures.

COMMON NAME Needle holder

CHARACTERISTICS Scissor blades are set behind the jaws. After the suture is tied into a knot, the surgeon can cut the suture material with the same instrument. This can speed up the time it takes to suture, but a false move can mean disaster, for it is possible that the surgeon may cut the suture material in the wrong place or inadvertently cut tissue. The lengths of this instrument can be 5½, 6½, or 7½ inches. They are also available with carbide jaws.

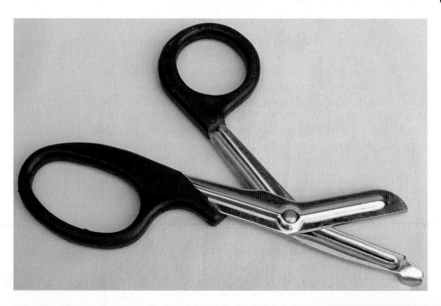

Economy/Utility Bandage Scissors

FUNCTION To remove bandages and other dressings.

CHARACTERISTICS These scissors are useful for removing large, bulky bandages, such as a Robert Jones bandage on a small animal or any bandage on a large animal. These scissors can also be used to cut tubing and thick bandaging materials.

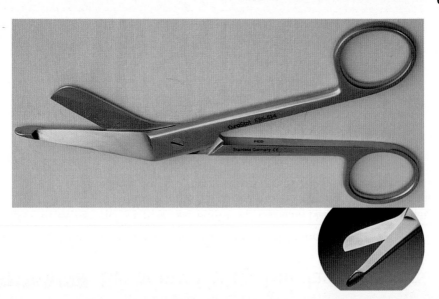

Lister Bandage Scissors

FUNCTION To remove bandages and other dressings.

CHARACTERISTICS One blade ends in a blunt triangle that is designed to push the skin out of the way as the tine is slipped under the bandage material, preventing accidental cutting of the skin by the scissors. The scissors are angled to allow users to get their fingers under the scissors and still be able to open and close them without being obstructed by the animal's body. The lengths range from 3½ to 8 inches.

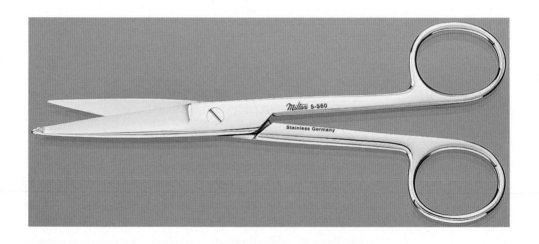

INSTRUMENT # Knowles Bandage Scissors

FUNCTION To remove bandages and other dressings.

CHARACTERISTICS The finer blades and straight or curved tines mean that the user can place them beneath tightly fitting bandages. Lengths range from 3½ to 8 inches.

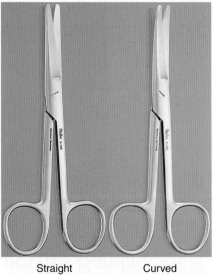

Straight   Curved

Mayo Scissors

FUNCTION To perform blunt dissection and to cut through bulky connective tissues.

CHARACTERISTICS These scissors have more mass than the Metzenbaum scissors and are commonly used for large animals. Lengths range from 5½ to 6¾ inches. Blades may be straight, curved, smooth, or serrated.

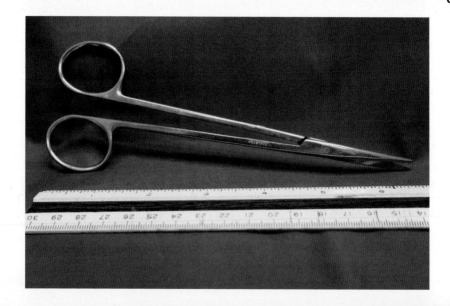

Metzenbaum Scissors

FUNCTION To blunt-dissect or cut soft tissues.

CHARACTERISTICS The fine blades on these scissors are approximately 1½ inches long and have blunt or pointed tips. Their lengths can be 4½, 5¾, or 7 to 11 inches, but the most common length is 7 inches. The blades can be straight or curved as well as smooth or serrated. These scissors should never be used to cut suture material or bandaging material because doing so dulls the blades. (Blunt dissection involves introducing the closed blades into an area; the blades are then opened and pulled backward through the tissues.) Blunt dissection stretches the small capillaries so they do not bleed, preventing the accidental cutting of tendons, ligaments, and large blood vessels.

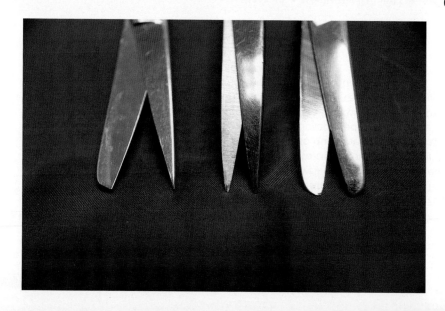

Operating Scissors—Sharp Blunt, Sharp Sharp, Blunt Blunt

FUNCTION To cut suture material or other inanimate materials.

CHARACTERISTICS Operating scissors are available in lengths of 4½, 5, 5½, and 6½ inches; the latter is the most common length. The tips of the blades are available in three combinations: the blunt-blunt scissors have blades that are rounded, the sharp-blunt scissors have one rounded and one pointed blade, and the sharp-sharp scissors have two blades that are pointed. The most common scissors of the three is the sharp blunt.

Operating Scissors—Sharp Blunt, Sharp Sharp, Blunt Blunt (continued)

NOTE
The tips are used to cut suture material, so they become dull rather quickly. If the scissors are to be sharpened, remind the sharpener to pay attention to the tips and to be careful not to grind them so much that they do not contact each other when the scissors are closed.

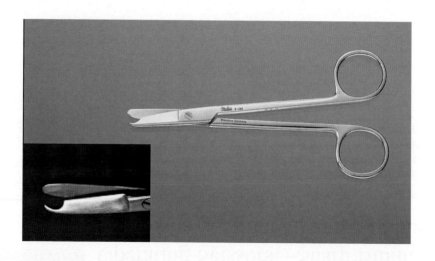

Straight Littauer Stitch Scissors

FUNCTION To remove sutures from an incision line or wound closure in large animals.

COMMON NAME Stitch scissors

CHARACTERISTICS These scissors are designed exactly like the Spencer delicate-stitch scissors but are larger at 4½ inches in length. Their size sometimes makes them difficult to use when removing sutures from small animals, but they can be used in a pinch.

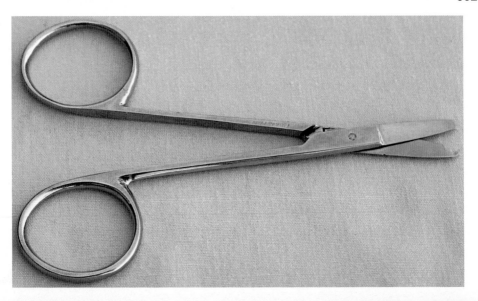

Straight Spencer Delicate-Stitch Scissors

FUNCTION To remove sutures from an incision line or wound closure in small animals.

COMMON NAME Stitch scissors

CHARACTERISTICS The tip of one blade of these scissors has a small depression that can be slipped between the suture material and the skin. The depression is just as sharp as the rest of the scissors and can cut the suture material with ease. These scissors are 3½ inches in length.

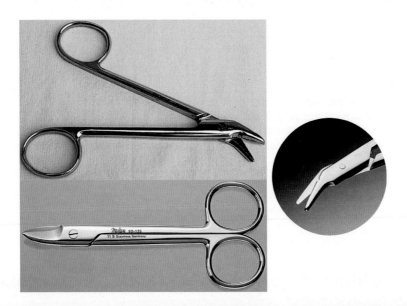

Wire Scissors

FUNCTION To cut stainless steel wire, which is commonly used in orthopedic surgery.

CHARACTERISTICS These scissors have short, compact, serrated blades. The serrations hold the wire in place, giving the scissors the ability to exert added pressure to cut heavier gauge wire without slipping or crimping the wire. The blades may be angled or straight, and the length is usually 4¾ inches.

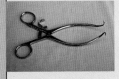

CHAPTER 18

Retractors and Rib Spreaders

Retractors are instruments that are used to hold open a wound, incision, or organs so that the surgeon can view the underlying tissues. Retractors are either handheld or self-retaining. Rib spreaders hold the ribs apart, allowing access to the thoracic cavity.

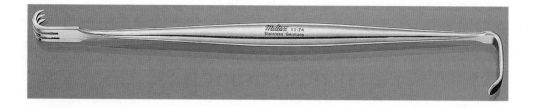

INSTRUMENT # Senn Rake Retractor

FUNCTION To hold open a wound or incision so that the surgeon can view the underlying tissues.

COMMON NAME Senns

CHARACTERISTICS This retractor is about 6¼ inches long and ends in three-pronged sharp or blunt points that curve sharply. It works well with smaller incisions and wounds than the US Army–pattern retractor. Small handles allow only one or two fingers to hold the instrument.

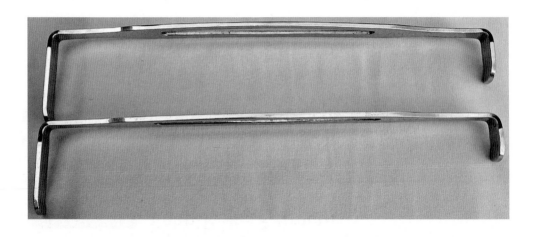

US Army Pattern Retractor

FUNCTION To hold open a wound or incision so that the surgeon can view the underlying tissues.

COMMON NAME Army retractor

CHARACTERISTICS This retractor comes in a set of two. It is a double-ended retractor with a lateral curve of the blades on each end. One end is a curved paddle about 5/8-inch wide and is placed over the wound edges to ease the wound open gently. The other end is angled and has longer ends to facilitate a good grip with the fingers or to go deeper into a wound cavity. The length of the retractor is 8½ inches.

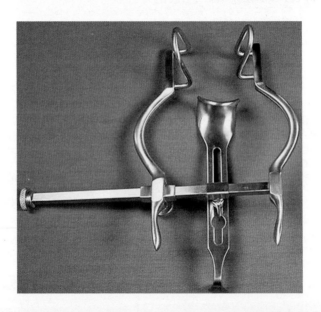

INSTRUMENT Balfour Retractor

FUNCTION To hold the abdominal wall open for the performance of surgical procedures.

CHARACTERISTICS Two wire-like blades are inserted into the incision line and spread apart. The scoop-like blade is positioned on the sternum or on the cranial aspect of the incision. All three blades can be adjusted to provide maximum exposure to the abdomen. The blades and the overall length of the Balfour retractor vary; there can be five different configurations to set this instrument for various surgical incisions.

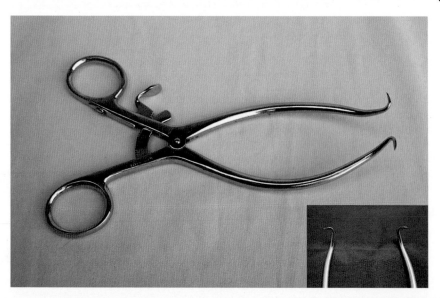

Gelpi Retractor

FUNCTION To maintain wound exposure during general surgery, orthopedic surgery, and neurosurgery.

CHARACTERISTICS Sharp, outward-curved points are arranged on a gently curved shaft that opens wider than the Weitlaner retractor. The length is usually 7 inches, although a "pedifine" Gelpi can be 3½, 4½, or 5½ inches long. It can also be purchased with stops on the points so that the tissue does not slide along the shafts.

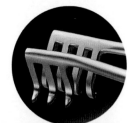

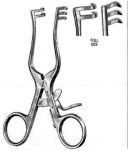

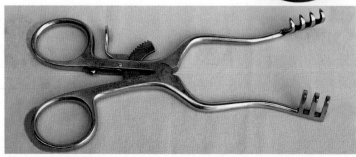

Weitlaner Retractor

FUNCTION To maintain muscle retraction during orthopedic surgery.

CHARACTERISTICS Sharp or blunt, outward-curved prongs are held open by a ratchet just above the handle. The prongs come in a 3 × 4 configuration. Lengths are 4, 5½, 6½, 8, and 9½ inches. The 4-inch retractor is referred to as a "baby Weitlaner"; its prongs are 2 × 3.

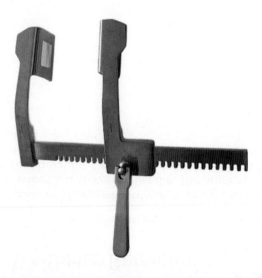

INSTRUMENT

Finochietto Rib Spreaders

FUNCTION To hold the ribs apart during thoracic surgery.

CHARACTERISTICS A heavy-duty rib spreader, the Finochietto has wide, square scoops that are positioned on long, thick shafts. To spread the scoops apart, the user turns a handle that is attached to one of the shafts. The spreader stays in position without a locking mechanism.

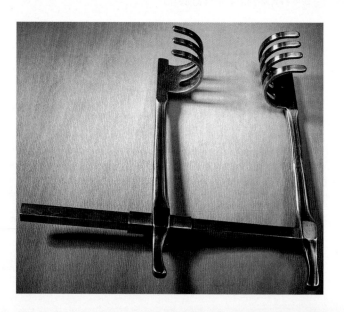

Frazier Rib Spreaders

FUNCTION To hold the ribs apart during thoracic surgery.

CHARACTERISTICS Half-curved, blunt prongs are positioned on the ribs and then pulled away from each other. The prongs are held in place by a turn screw. They are 3 × 4 and can be spread to 4 inches.

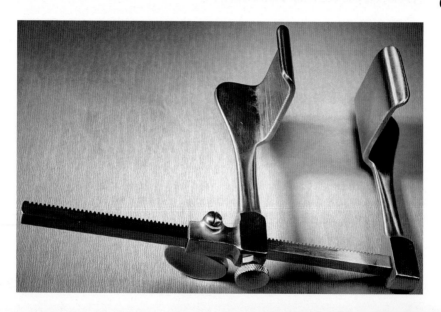

Tuffier Rib Spreader

FUNCTION To hold the ribs apart during thoracic surgery.

CHARACTERISTICS This rib spreader has solid square scoops that are positioned on short shafts. To spread the scoops apart, the user turns a dial attached to one of the shafts. The spreader is maintained in position by tightening the locking mechanism.

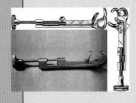

CHAPTER 19

Orthopedic Instruments

This chapter covers the standard instruments used in general orthopedic work. It is by no means a comprehensive list of instruments that an orthopedic surgeon may have available.

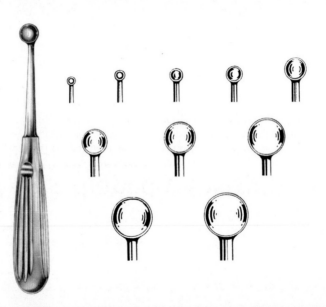

Bone Curette

FUNCTION To scrape out cancellous bone from the medullary cavity to perform bone grafts or to scrape osteochrondritis dissecans lesions.

CHARACTERISTICS One end is a cup with sharp edges; the other end is a wide handle. The cups may be oval or round. Lengths vary from 6½ to 8 inches. Cup sizes are indicated in two ways: in (ott) or O sizes as in suture material sizing or in millimeters. The Brun curette has one cup, while the Volkmann curette has one cup on each end.

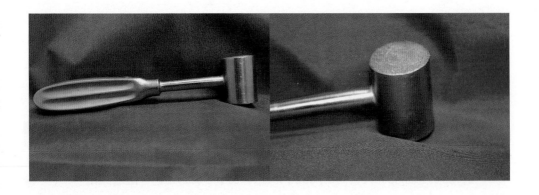

Bone Mallets

FUNCTION To set pins or to strike osteotomes or any other matter that requires pounding during surgery.

CHARACTERISTICS The heads of these mallets are filled with lead, making them heavy for their sizes. Lengths vary from 7½ to 8½ inches. They are known as Gerzog, Mead, and Lucae mallets and as the Richards combination mallet, which has a plastic-covered head on one side.

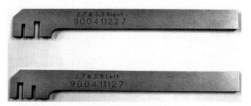

Bone bending irons

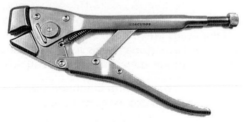

Bone bending pliers

Bone-Plate Bender

FUNCTION To bend plates to fit the contours of the bone being repaired.

CHARACTERISTICS One type is a straight, flat metal instrument with one or two grooves designed to cradle the plate while the surgeon applies pressure. The other type grips the plate between rollers and is bent when the surgeon closes the handles. The first type works well with small, narrow plates; the second type works with plates 3.5 mm and larger.

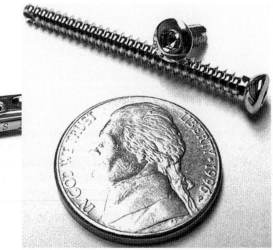

Bone plate

Bone screw

Bone Plates and Screws

FUNCTION To repair a fracture by applying a stainless-steel plate with stainless-steel screws or just stainless-steel screws.

CHARACTERISTICS Stainless-steel plates and screws come in a wide variety of sizes and styles. Most clinics have a number of them on hand.

694

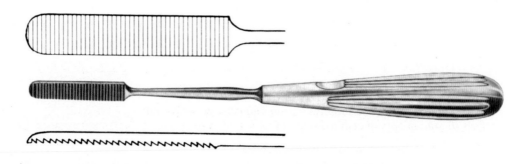

Bone Rasp

FUNCTION To smooth off rough edges of bones.

CHARACTERISTICS Raised crosshatches on the surface of this instrument look much like those on a file found on a carpenter's workbench. However, the end may be pointed, blunt, or rounded and may be flat or convex. Lengths range from 8½ to 11 inches. The instrument is also called a Putti or a Fomon rasp.

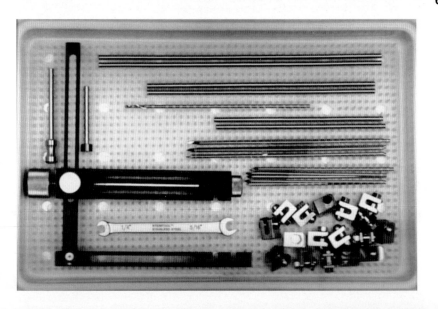

696

External Fixation Kits

FUNCTION To repair fractures by inserting pins into the bone from the outside.

CHARACTERISTICS A series of pins are inserted through the skin and into the bone. The pins are then connected to a connector rod, bringing the fracture into alignment.

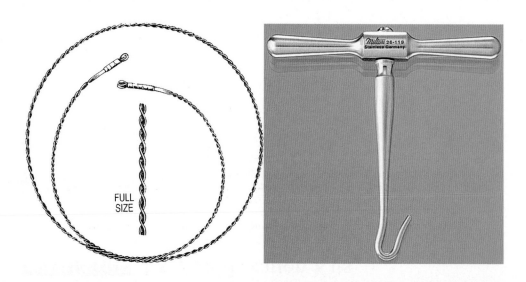

FULL
SIZE

698

Gigli Wire Saw and Handles

FUNCTION To cut through thick or heavy bone.

CHARACTERISTICS A rough wire is attached to or can be attached to handles. The wire is placed around a bone or horn, and a back-and-forth motion cuts through the matter with minimal effort.

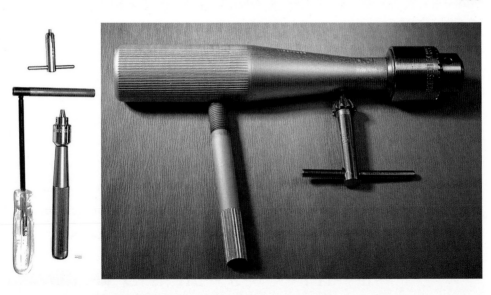

Intramedullary Pin Chuck

FUNCTION To place intramedullary pins into the bone.

CHARACTERISTICS This instrument has a chuck on one end that is the same as that found on an electric drill. It tightens down around the pin with the use of a key. It may have a solid handle or a hollow handle that allows the end of the pin to protrude. The latter type should have a detachable extension tube that covers the excess and protects surgeons from accidental injury or contamination by puncturing themselves or a glove with the pin tip. The Jacobs Hand Chuck has a blue handle.

702

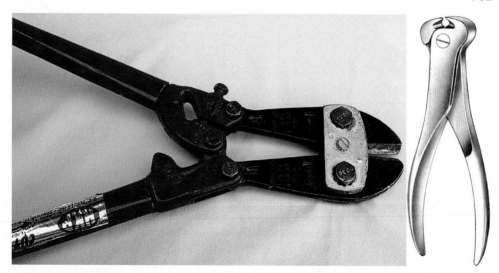

Pin cutter

Intramedullary Pin Cutter

FUNCTION To cut pins to the proper length.

CHARACTERISTICS Many models look much like bolt cutters. Thick jaws with spring action make cutting a stainless-steel pin easy work.

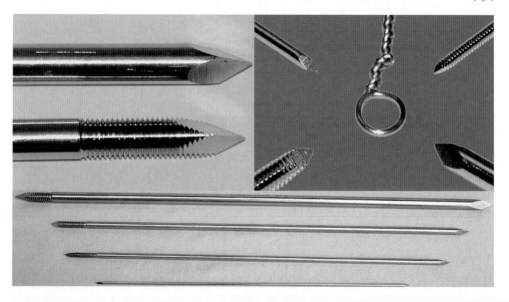

Intramedullary Pins

FUNCTION
To facilitate fracture stabilization by placing a stainless-steel rod in the medullary cavity.

CHARACTERISTICS
A stainless-steel rod has a sharp triangular point at one or both ends. The ends can be smooth or can be threaded on one or both ends. The ends are available in three different tips. A chisel (diamond) tip facilitates sliding the pin along the medullary cavity. A trocar point is considered a cutting tip, and the threaded trocar tip provides a solid anchor in the bone. A Steinmann pin has a trocar point on one end and is squared off on the other end. Pins come in lengths of 7 to 12 inches and 1/16 to 1/14 inches in diameter. The Kirschner wire/nail (K-wire) is also 7 to 12 inches long, but the diameters range from 0.035 to 0.625 mm.

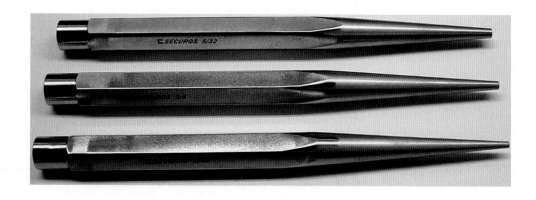

Intramedullary Pin Setter

FUNCTION To set an intramedullary pin into the medullary cavity.

CHARACTERISTICS Looking much like a punch, this instrument has an indented end that fits over the intramedullary pin; the other end has a handle that can withstand a blow by the bone mallet.

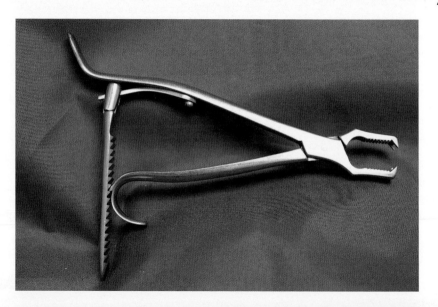

Kern Bone-Holding Forceps

FUNCTION To hold bone and bone fragments together for fixation with pins, screws, or plates. Care must be taken to avoid clamping this instrument too tightly because doing so can cause bruising to the bone.

CHARACTERISTICS The jaws are not as curved as those of the Lambert-Lowman clamp. They are held closed by a ratchet located at the bottom of the handles. Lengths range from 5¾ to 8½ inches, with or without the ratchet. The Lane bone-holding forceps looks very much like the Kern except that it has a greater jaw width and the length ranges from 13 to 17 inches.

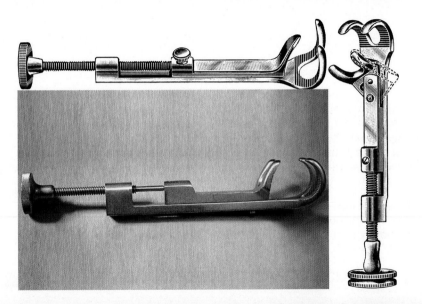

Lambert-Lowman Bone Clamp

FUNCTION   To hold bone and bone fragments together for fixation with pins, screws, or plates. The clamp does so without causing further trauma to the periosteum.

CHARACTERISTICS   Curved jaws sit at the top of a square handle with a knob at the bottom, which is used to bring the jaws together. The jaw configuration can be 1 × 1, 2 × 1, or 2 × 2. The instrument's length ranges between 4½ and 8 inches, and jaw lengths range from ¾ to 1½ inches. Some models allow the lower jaw to tilt.

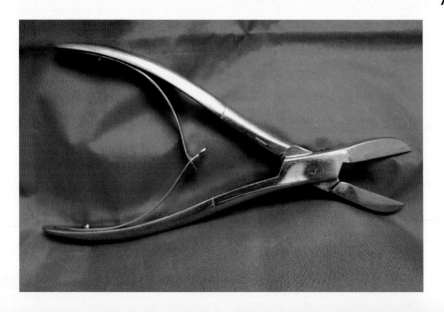

Liston Bone-Cutting Forceps

FUNCTION To cut bones.

CHARACTERISTICS This heavy-jawed instrument has smooth scissor-like jaws used to break ribs or other small bones. It is 5½ to 8 inches long and has straight or angled jaws. It is available with a double-action handle that increases the power of the instrument. A larger version of this instrument, called the Stille-Liston forceps, are available in 13 inches and the double-action handle is a standard feature.

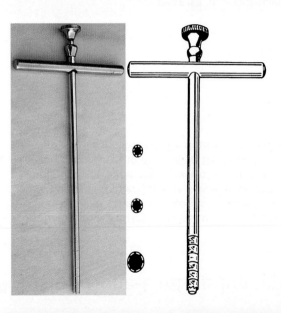

Michel Laminectomy Trephine

FUNCTION To perform bone biopsies or to drill small holes into the skull or sinus.

CHARACTERISTICS One end has small cutting blades that drill into the bone. The shaft has graduations for depth control, and there is a handle at the other end. The instrument is hollow and has a stylet to facilitate the capture of a biopsy. It is usually 7½ inches long.

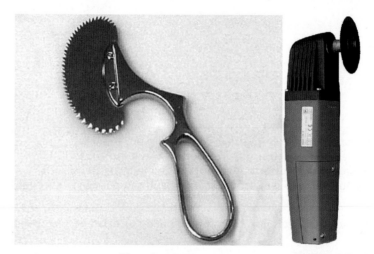

Manual cast saw   Electric cast saw

Orthopedic Cast Saw

FUNCTION To remove hard plaster or fiberglass casts.

CHARACTERISTICS This instrument can be hand operated for the removal of small casts or electrically powered for the removal of large, thick casts. Both instruments must be used with care when casting material is being removed.

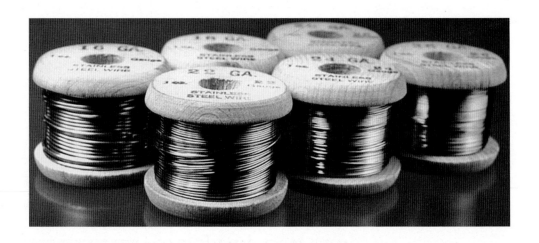

INSTRUMENT **Orthopedic Wire**

FUNCTION To repair fractures in combination with pins, plates, or external fixation apparatus.

CHARACTERISTICS A stainless-steel wire in 18-, 20-, and 22-gauge diameters is applied in a cerclage manner, which is similar to that of a twist tie.

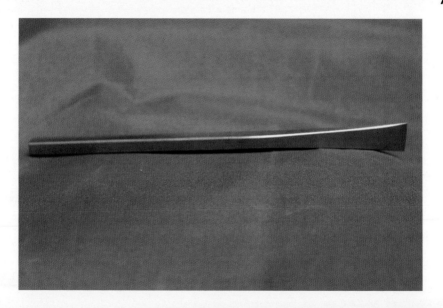

Osteotome

FUNCTION To cut through or to shape bone.

CHARACTERISTICS A tapered blade is situated at one end of a handle; the other end flares to accept the blow of a mallet. Osteotomes are 6½ to 9 inches long and vary in width from 6 to 38 mm. If the blade is curved, the instrument is called a gouge.

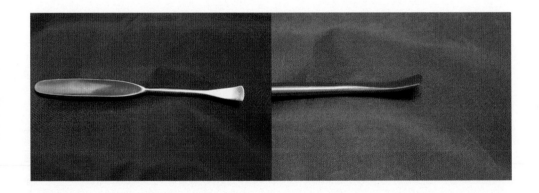

Periosteal Elevator

FUNCTION   To work under and lift the periosteum or soft tissues away from the bone.

CHARACTERISTICS   A curved bladelike end has a handle. It may be 6½ to 10 inches long and may have a blunt or a sharp blade that is scooped or curved. There may be a blade on each end of the handle.

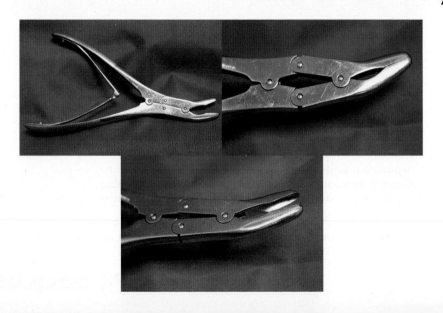

Ruskin Rongeur

FUNCTION To remove or break up small chunks of bone, cartilage, or fibrous tissue.

CHARACTERISTICS Small cups with sharp edges form the jaws of this instrument. It has double-action handles, giving it greater power when it is squeezed. It is 6 to 7¼ inches long and has jaw dimensions that range from 4 × 15- to 6 × 15-mm bites. The jaws can be angled or straight. They are also available with plain handles, which are commonly used on the smallest bones and are called Adson, Luer, or Lempert rongeurs.

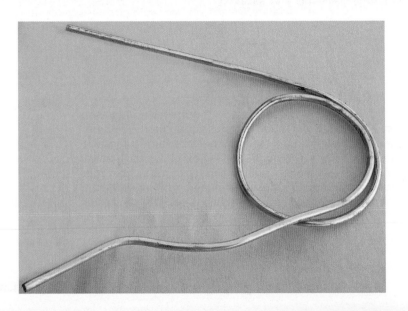

Splint Rod—Aluminum

FUNCTION To build a Thomas splint.

COMMON NAME Splint rod

CHARACTERISTICS Straight rods of various diameters can be bent into Thomas splints. Two sections are made; one section goes around the hip or shoulder, and the other goes beneath the foot. They are joined together with adhesive tape and can be adjusted based on the length of the limb.

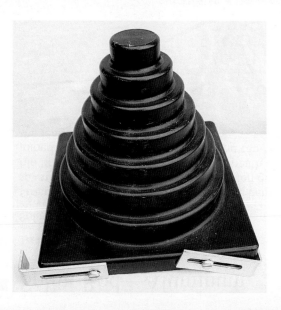

Splint-Rod Form

FUNCTION To make circular and angled bends in an aluminum rod to create a Thomas splint.

CHARACTERISTICS This form has a series of curved forms where an aluminum rod can be placed and then bent to form the necessary curves for a Thomas splint.

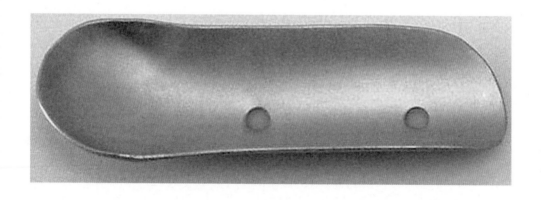

Splints—Mason Meta

FUNCTION To stabilize fractures of the digits, carpals, or metacarpals.

CHARACTERISTICS Aluminum or plastic material is shaped like an elongated spoon. These splints are available in a variety of lengths and widths so they can be fitted to a cat or dog of any size. The splint is held in place with adhesive tape. Extensions are available, and they are used to lengthen the splint.

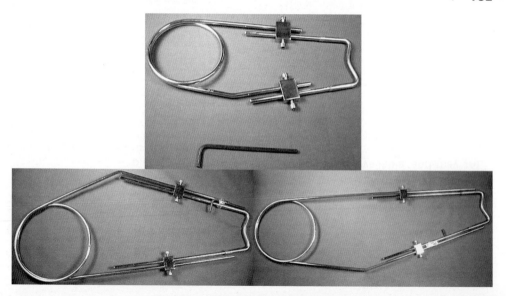

Splints—Thomas-Schroeder

FUNCTION To stabilize simple fractures of the lower leg bones, tibia and fibula, and radius and ulna.

CHARACTERISTICS An adjustable aluminum rod is shaped to fit a front or back leg. The circular area goes over the shoulder or hip to help keep the splint in place. The splint's length can be adjusted. The splint is strategically taped onto the animal to secure the fracture and to secure the splint to the animal.

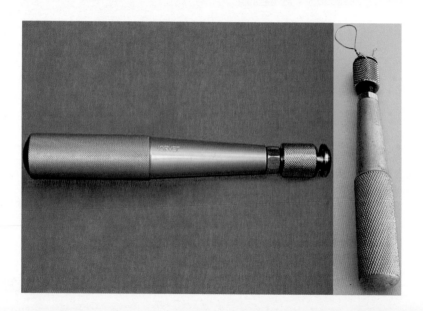

Wire Twister

FUNCTION To twist orthopedic wire to secure bone fragments.

CHARACTERISTICS A circular end has two holes for the insertion of the wire. Once the wire has been placed around the bone, the handle of the twister is turned, twisting down the wire in an orderly manner.

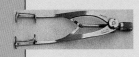

CHAPTER 20

Ophthalmic Instruments

This chapter covers instruments that are used in ophthalmic surgery and neurosurgery, but it is not a comprehensive list of the instruments that an ophthalmologist or neurosurgeon would have.

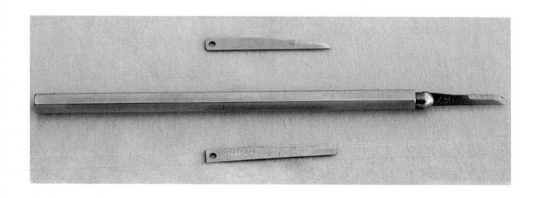

Beaver Surgical Blades—#64 and #67

FUNCTION To make incisions and other cuts during microsurgery.

CHARACTERISTICS These blades are shaped exactly like the #10 and #15, but they are much smaller.

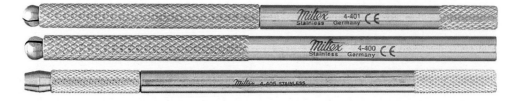

Beaver Surgical-Knife Handle

FUNCTION To hold a Beaver surgical blade.

CHARACTERISTICS A blade is attached to this instrument by turning the round end and opening a slit into which the blade is positioned. Turning the end to its closed position secures the blade in place.

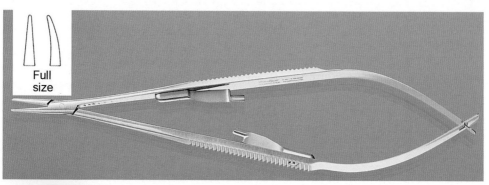

Full size

Castroviejo Needle Holder With Catch

FUNCTION To hold the fine suture needles required for placing sutures in an eye and performing neurosurgery.

CHARACTERISTICS Jaws that hold fine needles are attached to spring-loaded handles that catch or release with gentle pressure.

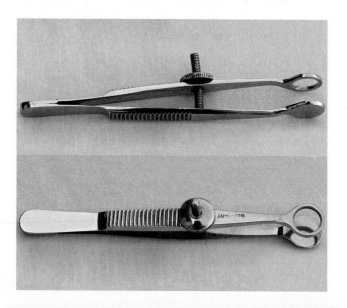

Chalazion Forceps

FUNCTION To isolate a chalazion (stye) for removal by stabilizing and everting the eyelid. They also provide hemostasis and a stable surface to excise the stye.

CHARACTERISTICS The ends of this instrument are both rounded and smooth. One side has a solid round panel, while the other end has an open circle. To bring the ends together, the user turns a small knob on the handle. The ends may be circular or oval, and the instrument may be straight or curved. Similar forceps are called Lambert, Ayers, Desmarres, and Hunt forceps.

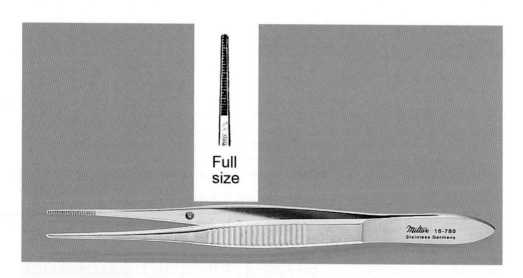

Full
size

Eye-Dressing Forceps

FUNCTION   To apply dressing materials to ophthalmic areas.

CHARACTERISTICS   These forceps look exactly like the dressing forceps found in regular surgical packs, but they are smaller and have finer jaws. They can cause trauma to tissues and should be used to handle only inanimate objects. They may be straight or curved, and sizes range from 4¾ to 6 inches.

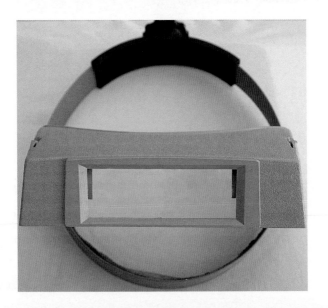

Eye Loupe

FUNCTION To magnify areas of concern; usually worn during microsurgery.

CHARACTERISTICS A plastic adjustable headband is fitted with magnifying glasses. Some models allow the lens to be propped up when normal vision is sufficient.

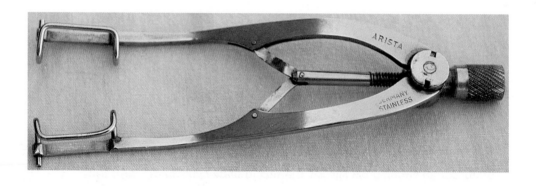

Eye Speculum

FUNCTION To hold the eyelids apart for ophthalmic examination or surgery.

CHARACTERISTICS Gently curved ends are designed to slide under each eyelid; a spring device or a turning knob spreads the eyelids apart. There are several versions of eye speculums: Castroviejo, Graefe, and Barraquer.

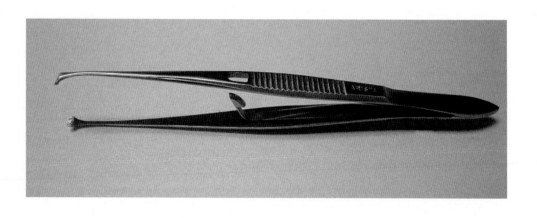

Graefe Eye-Fixation Forceps With Catch

FUNCTION To grasp and hold tissues in an atraumatic manner.

CHARACTERISTICS A combination of Allis tissue forceps and tissue forceps, the jaws of the Graefe forceps are configured like the Allis forceps and the handles are like the tissue forceps. The catch is designed to hold when the handles are pressed together; it is released by flicking the catch with a finger.

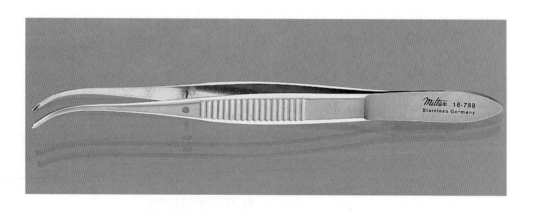

Half-Curved Tissue Forceps (1 × 2 Teeth)

FUNCTION To pick up tissue without causing trauma.

CHARACTERISTICS These forceps look exactly like the tissue forceps found in regular surgical packs but are smaller and have finer jaws. The structure of the teeth allows tissue to be picked up without causing trauma. They range in length from 4¾ to 6 inches, and the teeth in the jaws may be 1 × 2 or 2 × 3. The forceps may be straight or curved.

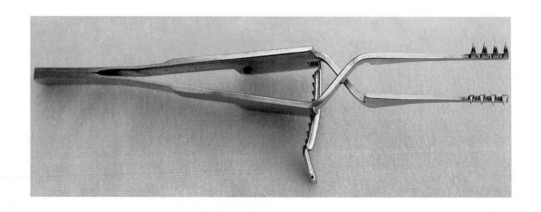

Holzheimer Retractor

FUNCTION To hold tissues apart so as to view underlying tissues or organs.

CHARACTERISTICS It is a 4-inch self-retaining retractor with a ratchet, and it has sharp outward-facing prongs. The user squeezes the handles to open the retractor, and the ratchet holds it open. Similar retractors are known as Alm, Jansen, and Allport retractors.

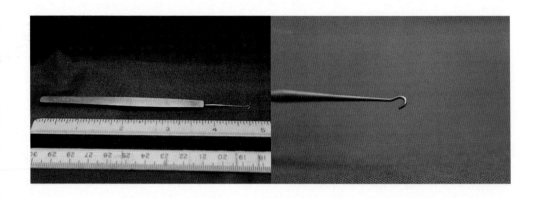

Iris Hook

FUNCTION To hold the iris in place during an ophthalmic procedure.

CHARACTERISTICS A tiny hook is situated at the end of a long handle. These hooks are also known as Tyrrell or Shepard hooks.

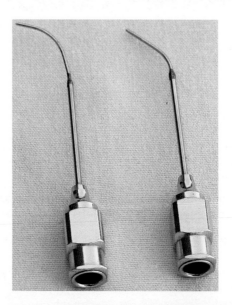

Lacrimal Cannula

FUNCTION To flush the lacrimal duct; it can also be used to flush the anal gland duct.

CHARACTERISTICS A regular aluminum hub and needle shaft has a copper tube attached to the end that tapers the diameter of the shaft down to 23- and 30-gauge diameters. The cannula is available with a straight or an angled shaft.

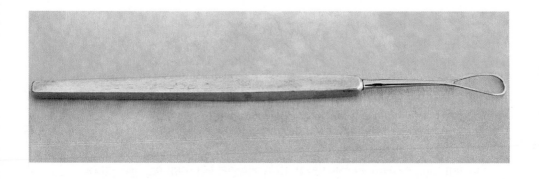

Lens Loop

FUNCTION To hold the lens in place during an ophthalmic procedure.

CHARACTERISTICS A circular or oval loop is situated at the end of a long handle.

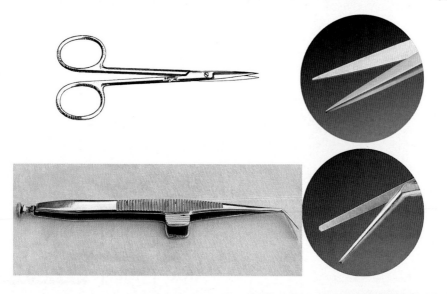

Scissors—Iris

FUNCTION To cut suture material and other nonviable materials.

CHARACTERISTICS The tips of these scissors look much like those of the operating scissors. The jaws are opened and closed by applying pressure to the spring handles. Some models have a standard scissors design. Tips can be found in the same combinations as those available for operating scissors.

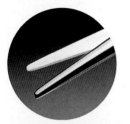

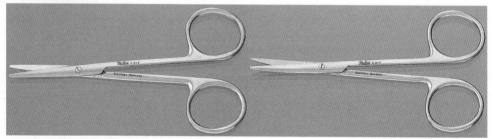

Straight   Curved

Scissors—Strabismus

FUNCTION To cut delicate tissues and perform blunt dissection.

CHARACTERISTICS These scissors look much like the Metzenbaum scissors but are more delicate. Their lengths range between 4 and 5½ inches; the blades may be curved or straight.

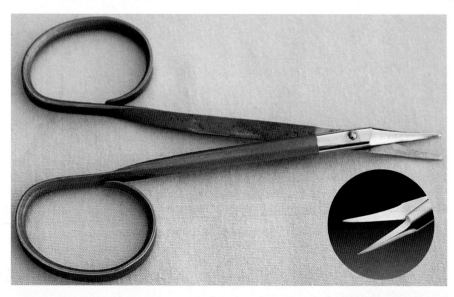

INSTRUMENT   Scissors—Tenotomy

FUNCTION   To divide and dissect the muscles and tendons of the eye during recession and resection for strabismus surgery.

CHARACTERISTICS   Short, blunt, narrowed tips are straight or slightly curved and have a small handle. The length of the scissors is 4½ inches. The most common names for these scissors are Stevens, Ribbon Stevens, and Westcott.

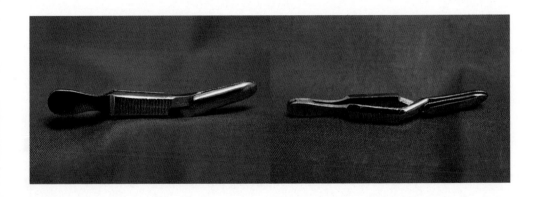

Serrefine

FUNCTION To hold and crush tissues, occlude small vessels, or to tag and hold bridle or fine sutures.

COMMON NAME Bulldog clamp

CHARACTERISTICS The jaws are similar to those of the other hemostatic forceps and also may be straight or curved. They function when the handles are squeezed, opening the jaws in a crossover motion. Similar forceps are known as Dieffenbach, DeBakey, Glover, and Johns Hopkins forceps.

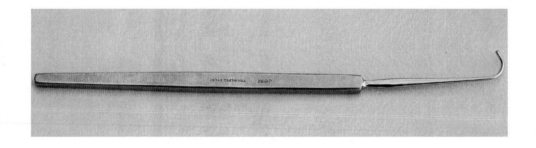

Strabismus Hook

FUNCTION To hook or stabilize the muscles surrounding the eyes.

CHARACTERISTICS A blunt-ended hook is situated at the end of a long handle. These hooks are known as Graefe or Jameson hooks.

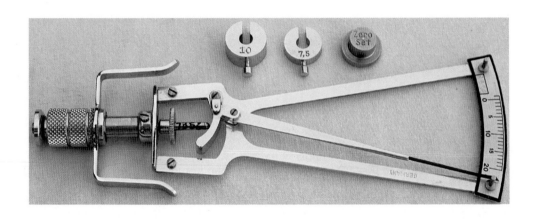

Tonometer

FUNCTION To measure intraocular pressure.

CHARACTERISTICS One end of this instrument is placed on the surface of the eye; this engages a small needle gauge that measures the ocular pressure in the eye. Small weights included with the tonometer measure whether the pressure is higher than the original setting on the gauge.

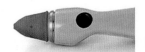

Disposable protective film over tip

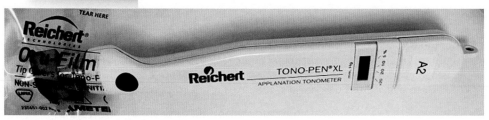

Tono-Pen

FUNCTION To measure intraocular pressure.

CHARACTERISTICS The end of this instrument is placed on the surface of the eye; this engages a pressure plate that measures the ocular pressure of the eye. The pressure is displayed in a digital window.

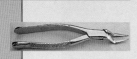

CHAPTER 21

Dental Instruments

This chapter covers dental instruments that are used in most routine dental cleaning. However, this is not a comprehensive list of all the dental instruments available.

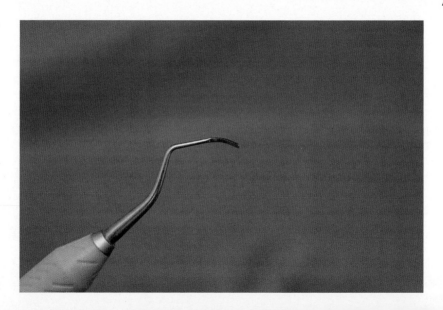

Barnhart Curettes—½

FUNCTION To remove tartar from the subgingival and supragingival surfaces of teeth.

CHARACTERISTICS The Barnhart curettes are used on the buccal and lingual surfaces posterior teeth as well as other teeth in the mouth. They have a long shank and thin blade. The ends are designed to be flipped from one end to the other as you move from buccal to lingual surfaces.

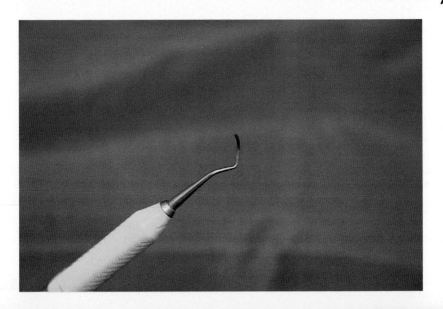

Columbia Universal Curettes—13/14

FUNCTION To remove tartar from the subgingival and supragingival surfaces of teeth.

CHARACTERISTICS Curettes are used on the buccal and lingual surfaces or the anterior and posterior teeth. They have a short shank with a medium to thin blade. The ends are designed to be flipped from one end to the other as you move from buccal to lingual surfaces.

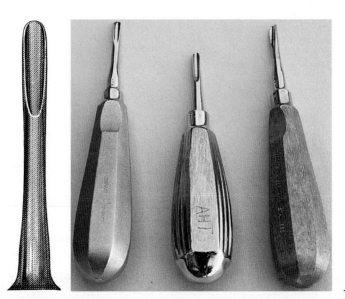
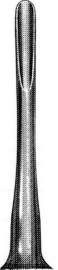

Dental Elevators

FUNCTION To loosen a tooth from the periodontal ligament before its extraction.

CHARACTERISTICS These elevators have pockets of various shapes to fit the surface of a particular tooth and various lengths to accommodate various teeth.

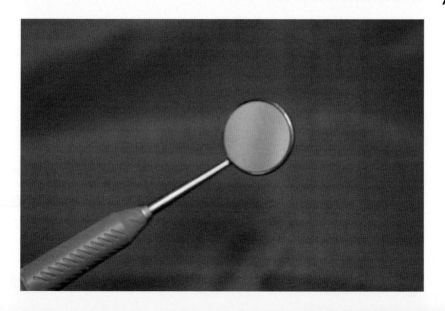

Dental Mirror

FUNCTION   To view and illuminate difficult to see tooth surfaces in the mouth.

CHARACTERISTICS   The mirror is moved about the mouth on the lingual or palette surfaces and is also used as a buccal retractor to view those surfaces.

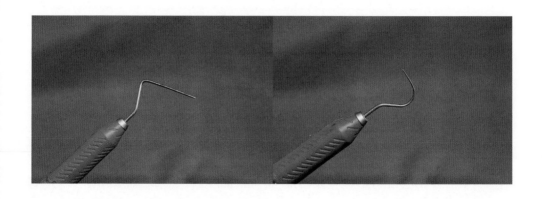

Depth Probe and Explorer

FUNCTION The probe used to examine teeth for depth of the sulci or periodontal pocket. The explorer evaluates surface irregularities, caries, and tartar detection, furcation involvement, and exploration of pockets.

CHARACTERISTICS The explorer end has a blunt tip and graduations that are measured in millimeters; it is placed into the sulcus on the long axis of the tooth to measure the depth of the pocket. The probe end is half curved and ends in a fine point. It is dragged across the surface of the tooth to check for missed tartar, while the pointed end is used to check for soft spots.

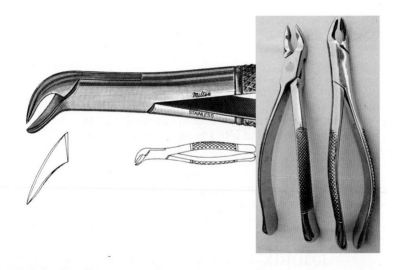

Incisor-, Canine-, and Premolar-Extracting Forceps

FUNCTION To aid in the removal of the incisor, canine, and premolar teeth.

CHARACTERISTICS The jaws on this extracting forceps have deeper indentations to accommodate larger teeth; the handles are slightly bent to facilitate the removal of teeth.

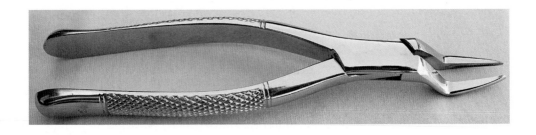

Incisor- and Root-Extracting Forceps

FUNCTION To grasp the small incisor or the root of a tooth that is to be removed.

CHARACTERISTICS Fine jaws have small indentations on a handle that is almost straight.

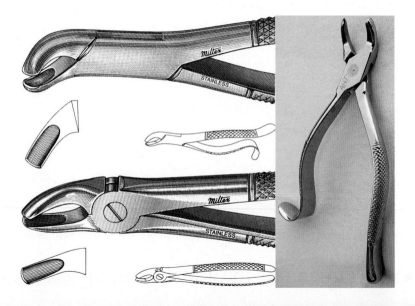

794

Molar-Extracting Forceps

FUNCTION To aid in the removal of molars.

CHARACTERISTICS The jaws of these forceps are very deep, and the handles are usually sharply angled to allow access to the tooth and facilitate its removal.

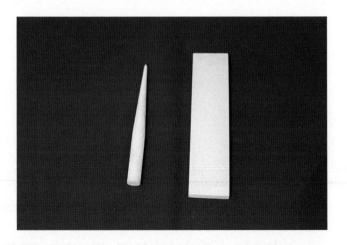

Sharpening Stones

FUNCTION To sharpen tartar scrapers and curettes

CHARACTERISTICS The flat stone and conical stone are used to sharpen tartar scrapers, usually using a drop of water or oil. There are many videos online that demonstrate the technique.

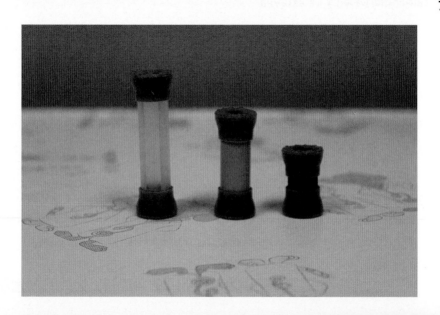

Smart Veterinary Mouth Gag Set

FUNCTION To hold open the mouth of a small animal.

CHARACTERISTICS This set of six mouth gags is used on canine teeth. They are designed to not overextend the jaw, which can cause injury to those tissues. The smallest sizes are recommended for felines. They can be sterilized by gas or steam autoclaves, and their sturdy design allows them to be used many times.

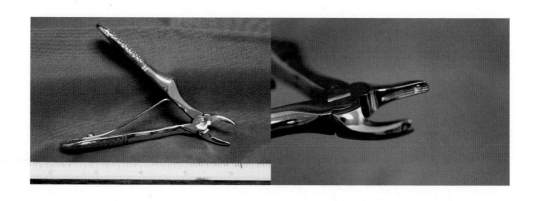

Tartar-Removing Forceps

FUNCTION To remove tartar from the supragingival surfaces of teeth.

CHARACTERISTICS The tartar-removing forceps are used to quickly break up accumulations of tartar on the tooth surfaces. Many of them have one bent jaw as well as the one pictured here. Care must be taken to not apply excess pressure to twist while applying pressure to break the tartar.

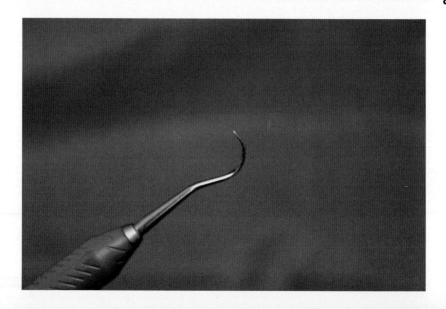

Tartar Scalers—Jacquette

FUNCTION To remove tartar and plaque from the supragingival surfaces of teeth.

CHARACTERISTICS The Jacquette 33 scaler is used interproximally on the anterior teeth. Jacquette scaler H5 is used interproximally on the posterior teeth.

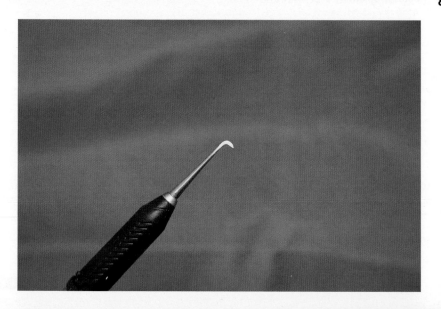

Tartar Scaler Morse 0-00

FUNCTION To remove tartar and plaque from the supragingival surfaces of teeth.

CHARACTERISTICS This thin blade is at a 90-degree angle designed for supragingival scaling of crowded or overlapping teeth and is also used for stain removal.

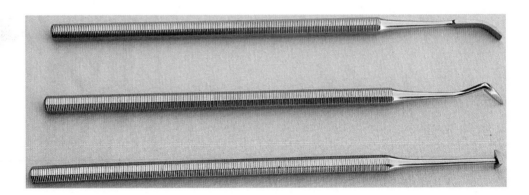

Tartar Scrapers—Single Ended

FUNCTION To remove tartar and plaque from the surfaces of teeth.

CHARACTERISTICS These scrapers are available in a variety of shapes and angles that fit specific teeth.

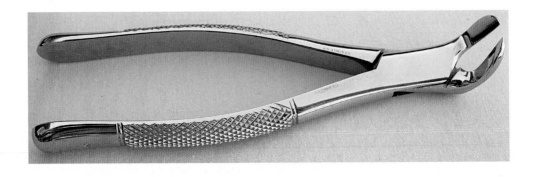

Tooth-Splitting and Separating Forceps

FUNCTION To split multirooted teeth for removal.

CHARACTERISTICS These flat, sharply angled forceps provide maximal torque to split a tooth.

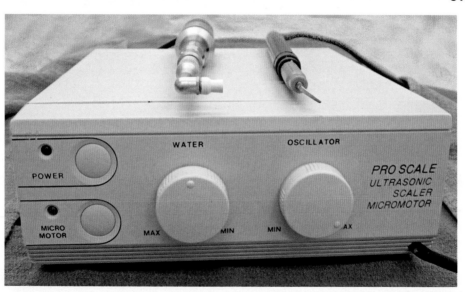

Dental Cavitron With Polisher

FUNCTION To remove tartar from teeth and then polish them so they are smooth.

CHARACTERISTICS Ultrasonic motion removes tartar with a handpiece and heads that are angled to conform to a tooth's surface. The unit requires water to keep the teeth cool; otherwise, they would be damaged by the heat created by the high-speed ultrasonic motion. The polisher is usually a separate handpiece. It uses a paste like a polishing compound that smooths the tooth surface so as to eliminate grooves caused by hand and ultrasonic scaling. The polisher operates at high speeds and can cause heat damage to the tooth. It is imperative to use polishing paste and to touch the tooth surface for only a second or two before moving on to the next tooth.

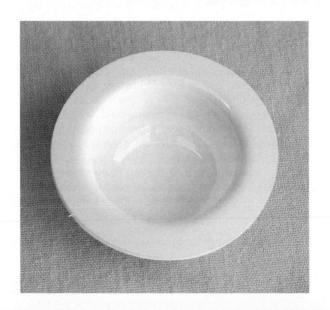

Prophy Paste Cups

FUNCTION To hold the polish used to smooth the surface of the tooth.

CHARACTERISTICS A small plastic cup. It may be disposable or may be attached to a ring and reused.

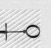

CHAPTER 22

Teat Instruments

This chapter covers instruments that are used in cattle, especially dairy cattle, to correct defects and problems with teats.

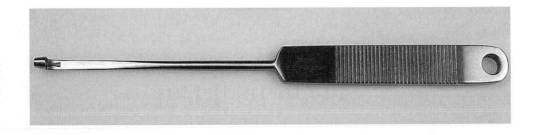

Cornell Teat Curette

FUNCTION   To scrape the inside of the teat canal and remove obstructions or tumors or to take biopsy specimens.

CHARACTERISTICS   The bottom of the loop has a sharp edge and is affixed to a handle. The loop gathers tissue as it is pulled out of the teat.

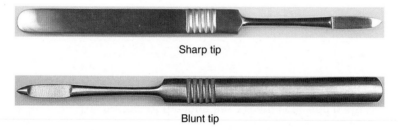

Sharp tip

Blunt tip

Lichty Teat Knife or Bistoury

FUNCTION To open stenotic teats by incising through scar tissue or other constricting tissue.

CHARACTERISTICS A slim stainless-steel blade is attached to a handle. The point or tip of the blade may be sharp or blunt.

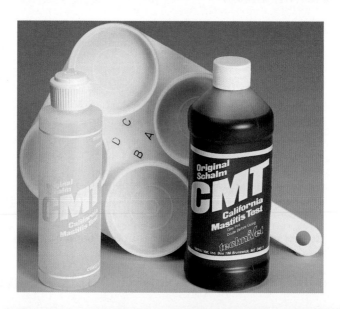

Mastitis Test Kit

FUNCTION To screen for and diagnose mastitis in cattle.

CHARACTERISTICS The paddle is divided into four quarters that correspond to the four teats. Milk from each quarter is placed into its corresponding circle. A reagent is mixed with the milk, and if agglutination is seen, mastitis is suspected.

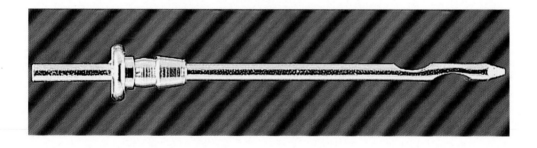

Milking Tubes

FUNCTION To keep an injured teat, open for milking.

CHARACTERISTICS These tubes are inserted after surgery or after an injury that may cause the teat to swell. They help to keep the canal patent while the teat heals.

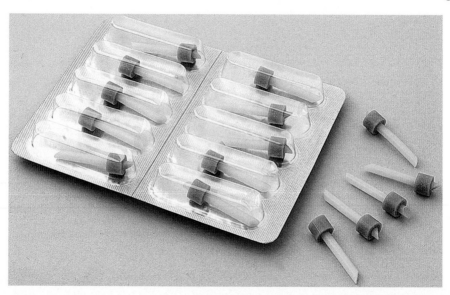

Teat Dilator

FUNCTION To open the teat canal.

CHARACTERISTICS A gradually widening instrument is slipped into the teat canal to open it.

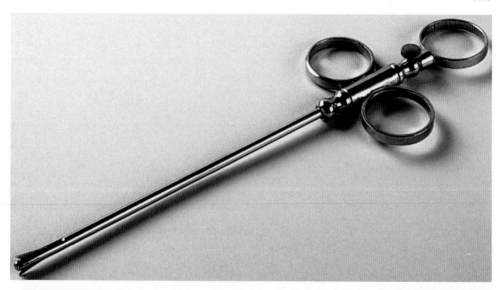

Teat Slitter

FUNCTION   To make an incision from the inside to the outside.

CHARACTERISTICS   The blade of this slim instrument is hidden inside the shaft. The instrument is slipped into the teat canal, and the blade is released by pushing on the ring; this allows an incision to be made from the inside to the outside.

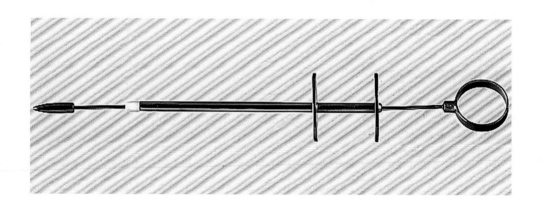

Teat Tumor Extractor

FUNCTION To remove tumors or other fibrous material from the teat canal.

CHARACTERISTICS A bullet-shaped tip is slender enough to be introduced into the teat canal. The base of the bullet tip is sharp and will slice through the tumor in the teat canal. The instrument is slid into the teat canal bypassing the tumor. The plunger on the instrument is pushed and as the instrument is removed from the teat canal, the sharp blades remove the tumor tissue.

PUSHED AND AS THE INSTRUMENT IS REMOVED FROM THE CANAL.

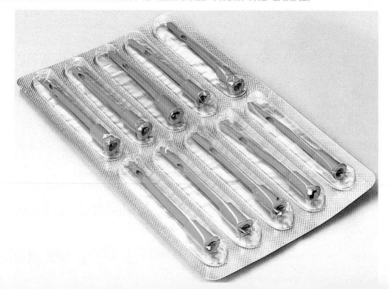

INSTRUMENT Udder Infusion Cannula

FUNCTION To administer medications into the teat canal. Other possible uses include draining a quarter with mastitis, keeping a teat canal or sphincter open during and after surgery, flushing an abscess, and performing a peritoneal tap.

CHARACTERISTICS A blunted needle-like tube can be inserted into the teat canal by using a syringe, medication can then be injected.

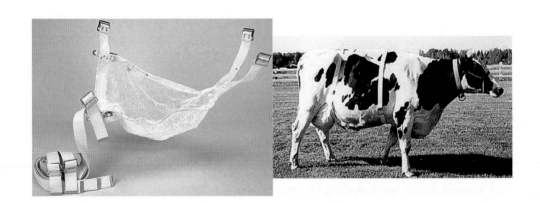

Udder Support

FUNCTION To support an injured or pendulous udder.

CHARACTERISTICS A net is placed around the udder and then strapped to the cow's body. This transfers the weight of the udder to the cow's back and keeps the udder from being stepped on or injured.

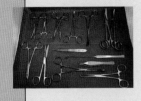

CHAPTER 23

Surgical Instrument Packs

The following list of surgical instruments is often packed together and sterilized by veterinary technicians. Each veterinarian has their own preference for what goes into a particular pack. For example, some veterinarians like curved forceps, while others like straight forceps. The following lists have been kept general in nature and can be interchanged with other instruments of choice. *These pages can also be utilized as a self-quiz. Try to identify the instruments you have already learned about in the preceding pages and then check the list on the following to page to see how well you did.*

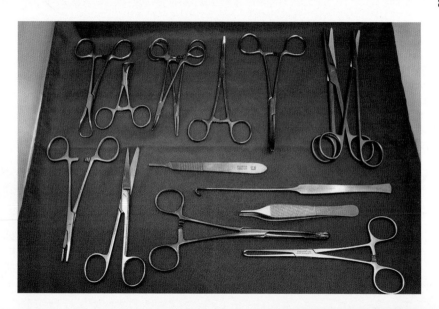

Instruments in the table below correspond to the photo above and are in order from left to right starting at the top.

Spay (Ovariohysterectomy) Packs

Table 23.1 Canine/Feline

Quantity	Instrument	Chapter Photo Reference
2	Backhaus towel forceps—5.5″	15
4	Backhaus towel forceps—3.5″ or Jones towel forceps	15
2–4	Halsted mosquito forceps—curved or straight	15
2	Kelly forceps or Crile forceps—curved or straight	15
2–4	Rochester Carmalt forceps—curved or straight	15

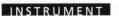
Spay (Ovariohysterectomy) Packs (continued)

1	Metzenbaum and/or Mayo scissors	17
1	Olsen-Hegar or Mayo-Hegar needle holder	17
1	Operating scissors—sharp-blunt, sharp-sharp, blunt-blunt	17
1	#3 Scalpel handle	16
1	Snook's ovariectomy hook	16
1	Adson-Brown tissue forceps	15
1	Allis tissue forceps	15
1	Foerster sponge-holding forceps	165
*1	Groove director—optional	16

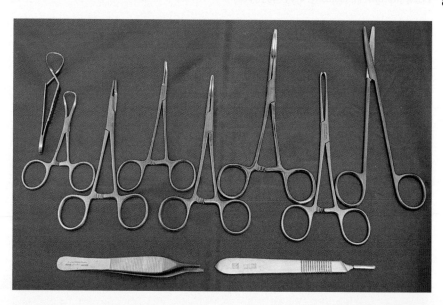

Instruments in the table below correspond to the photo above and are in order from left to right starting at the top.

INSTRUMENT

Neuter (Orchiectomy) Surgical Pack

Table 23.2 Canine

Quantity	Instrument	Chapter Photo Reference
4	Jones towel forceps—3.5″ or Backhaus towel forceps	15
1	Olsen-Hegar or Mayo-Hegar needle holder	17
2	Halsted mosquito forceps—curved or straight	15

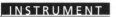

2	Kelly forceps or Crile forceps—curved or straight	15
2	Rochester Carmalt forceps—curved or straight	15
1	Allis tissue forceps	15
1	Metzenbaum and/or Mayo scissors	17
1	Adson-Brown tissue forceps	15
1	#3 Scalpel handle	16

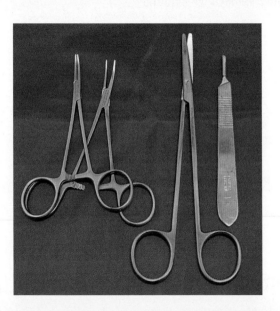

Instruments in the table below correspond to the photo above and are in order from left to right starting at the top.

Neuter (Orchiectomy) Surgical Pack

Table 23.3 Feline

Quantity	Instrument	Chapter Photo Reference
2	Halsted mosquito forceps—curved or straight	15
1	Metzenbaum scissors	17
1	#3 Scalpel handle	16

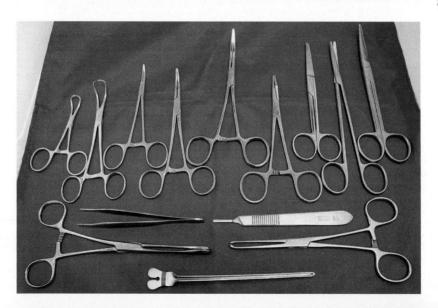

Instruments in the table below correspond to the photo above and are in order from left to right starting at the top.

General Surgical Pack—All Species

Quantity	Instrument	Chapter Photo Reference
4	Backhaus towel forceps—3.5" or (Jones towel forceps—not pictured)	15
2	Backhaus towel forceps—5.5"	15
2–4	Halsted mosquito forceps—curved or straight	15
2	Kelly forceps or Crile forceps—curved or straight	15

General Surgical Pack—All Species (continued)

4	Rochester Carmalt forceps—curved or straight	15
1	Olsen-Hegar or Mayo-Hegar needle holder	17
1	Operating scissors—sharp-blunt, sharp-sharp or blunt-blunt	17
1	Metzenbaum and/or Mayo scissors	17
1	Adson-Brown tissue forceps	15
1	#3 Scalpel handle	16
1	Foerster sponge-holding forceps	15
1	Allis tissue forceps	15
*1	Groove director—optional	16

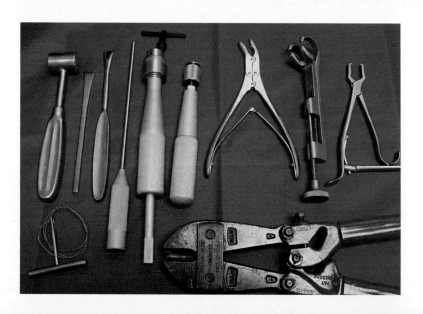

Instruments in the table below correspond to the photo above and are in order from left to right starting at the top.

Orthopedic Surgical Pack

Quantity	Instrument	Chapter Photo Reference
1	Bone mallet	19
1	Osteotome	19
1	Periodontal elevator	19
1	Intramedullary pin setter	19
1	Intramedullary pin chuck	19
1	Wire twister	19
1	Ruskin rongeur	19
1	Lambert-Lowman or Kern bone-holding forceps	19

Orthopedic Surgical Pack (continued)

Quantity	Instrument	Chapter Photo Reference
1	Gigli wire saw with handles	19
1	Intramedullary pin cutter	19

Ancillary Orthopedic Instruments—Usually packed and sterilized as singles or in groups and separately from the general orthopedic instruments. Photos of these can be found in Chapter 19. Examples of these separate packs include:

- Intramedullary pins—assorted sizes—usually two of each
- Orthopedic wire—one or more sizes
- Bone plate and screws kits
- External fixation kits

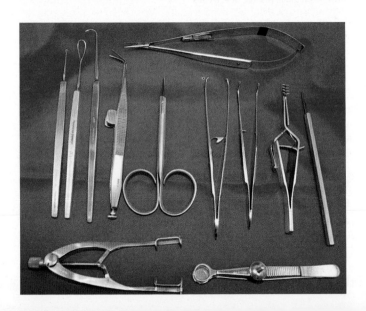

Instruments in the table below correspond to the photo above and are in order from left to right starting at the top.

INSTRUMENT # Ophthalmic Surgical Instruments

Quantity	Instrument	Chapter Photo Reference
1	Castroviejo needle holder (across the top)	20
1	Iris hook	20
1	Lewis lens loop	20
1	Strabismus hook	20
1	Iris scissors	20
1	Tenotomy scissors	20

1	Graefe eye-fixation forceps with catch	20
1	Half-curved tissue forceps 1 × 2 teeth	20
1	Holzheimer retractor	20
1	Beaver surgical knife handle (microblade)	20
1	Eye speculum	20
1	Chalazion forceps	20
Optional	Serrefine	20

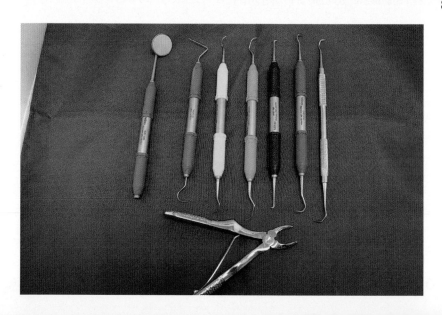

Instruments in the table below correspond to the photo above and are in order starting at the upper left.

INSTRUMENT # Dental Prophylaxis Kit

Quantity	Instrument	Chapter Photo Reference
1	Dental mirror	21
1	Depth probe and explorer	21
1	Columbia 12/14 universal curette	21
1	Barnhart 1–2 curette	21
1	Morse scaler 0-00 or	21
1	Jacquette scaler 33/H5	21
1	Gracey posterior/anterior scaler	21
1	Tartar removing forceps	21

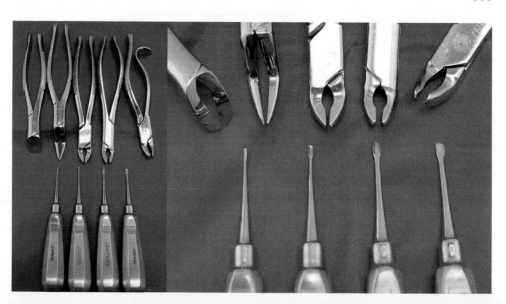

Instruments in the table below correspond to the photo above and are in order from left to right starting at the top.

Dental Periodontal Extraction Kit

Quantity	Instrument	Chapter Photo Reference
1	Tooth splitting and separating forceps	21
1	Incisor-root extracting forceps	21
2	Incisor-, canine-, and premolar-extracting forceps	21
1	Molar extracting forceps	21
1 each	Periodontal elevators—sizes A–D	21

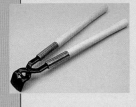

Care of Instruments

Surgical instruments are designed to correct physical problems that require surgery. When a good-quality surgical instrument is used for the right job, that instrument should last a lifetime. That life can be extended if, during that use, it is cleaned and maintained properly.

New Instrument Inspection Checklist

- Inspect each instrument to ascertain that it is in good shape. If it is defective, return it to the company for an exchange or refund. Any instrument that does not meet the following standards should be rejected. It is also a good idea to check in-use instruments as they are cleaned to catch worn out instruments.
- Check for roughness or pitting of the surface. If any such defects exist, corrosion, rusting, and staining are usually the next developments.
- If there are moving parts, check for smoothness of engaging and disengaging and for proper meshing of the jaws.
- If two parts of an instrument are held together by a screw, the screw should be tight.

Tests for Specific Instruments

- Hemostats: Clamp the box lock of a hemostat at the first tooth, it should produce an audible snap as it engages.
  Reverse the jaws and tap the handles on the palm of your hand, the box lock should not spring open.
- Scissors: Check for sharpness. Cut through four layers of gauze with just the tips of the blades. They should cut cleanly.
- Scissors shorter than 4 inches are tested with no fewer than two layers.
- Needle holders are checked by clamping an ordinary suture needle into their jaws, to the second tooth on the box lock. It should not be possible to turn the needle with one's fingers.

Cleaning Instruments

Soiled instruments must be cleaned as soon as possible after use. Within 10 minutes, blood or tissue left on an instrument starts to break down the instrument's surface, causing stains, pitting, or rusting. If instruments cannot be cleaned within that time frame, they should be kept moist by being placed in a wet towel; however, they should not be soaked, because that only hastens the breakdown of instruments.

- Detergents and solutions used for cleaning instruments must have a pH of 7 or 8.5 and diluted properly to prevent instrument breakdown.
- Initially clean with a scrub brush and cleanser or an ultrasonic cleaner with a cleanser. Scrub brushes should be designed specifically for medical instruments. Too hard a bristle can cause damage and fail to get into the cracks and crevices.
  - All the instruments in a pack are to be cleaned, even if they have not been used.

- Hand Cleaning
  - Open all the jaws and place in the cleaning solution.
  - Scrub each instrument with attention to the grooves in the jaws, box locks, and joints.
  - Rinse in water (distilled water is recommended) and dry thoroughly. Pay attention to box locks, joints, and moving parts.
  - Lubricate, all moving parts with a specially designed lubricant for surgical instruments.
- Ultrasonic Cleaning
  - Ultrasonic cleaners (see Chapter 14) provide rapid and thorough cleaning of surgical instruments. They work by producing bubbles that implode against the instrument, "blasting" the debris from the surface, and cleaning in places where brushes cannot reach.
  - Clean the obvious debris from the instruments with a brush and rinse.

- Separate instruments into two groups: sharp and nonsharp. Then separate them according to the type of material, such as brass, stainless steel, and so forth.
- Open all box locks, and any instrument designed to be taken apart should be separated.
- Place the instruments in the provided basket without overfilling it.
- Fill the ultrasonic cleaner with detergent designed for the ultrasonic cleaner at the proper dilution. Do not use regular detergent as the ultrasonic cleaner will overflow with bubbles!
- Set the timer for 10 to 15 minutes.
- Remove the tray promptly after the timer has gone off, and rinse thoroughly with distilled water.
- Carefully dry and lubricate instruments. Then store properly or regroup instruments and pack into the various surgical packs.

Causes of Instrument Breakdown

The top three causes of breakdown are tap water, surgical wraps, and moisture.

- The water source for an autoclave can be an instrument killer. Tap water contains minerals that, when vaporized, become concentrated and form layers on instruments. As the instruments dry, the minerals cause pitting and corrosion. Always use distilled water in the autoclave to prevent the buildup of minerals. If an autoclave is supplied by a direct water line, it is important to check the owner's manual for instructions on cleaning the steam-line filter.
- Surgical wraps laundered with everyday detergents are alkaline based, and most washing machines do not rinse well enough to remove the metallic ions that remain in the wrap material. The instruments wrapped in these fabrics and autoclaved vaporize the metallic ions deposited on the instruments. For this reason,

autoclaves must be cleaned on a weekly basis to prevent the buildup of these minerals and metallic ions, and surgical wraps should be put through two rinse cycles. It is also advisable to avoid overloading the washing machine when cleaning surgical wraps to ensure clean, well-rinsed wraps. Moisture damage can occur, if the autoclave is not allowed to go through the drying cycle and if the instrument packs are not allowed to dry on a rack before being stored. Wrapped surgical packs can develop condensation, which not only contaminates the pack but also causes the instruments to rust or corrode.

- Soaking instruments in cold sterilization solutions for extended periods can also cause rusting unless a rust-prohibitor sterilizing solution is being used.

Appendix A

Advanced Monitors Corporation
7098 Miratech Dr. Ste. 130
San Diego, California
Phone: 877-838-8367
Website: www.pet-temp.com

Allflex/Merk Animal Health
2805 E 14th
DFW Airport, Texas
Phone: 800-989-8247
Website: allflexusa.com

Arrowquip
Phone: 866-383-7827
Website: www.arrowquip.com
Email: cs@arrowquip.com

Bella VMS
Phone: 403-231-3366
Website: bellavms.com
Email: info@bellavms.com

Berkelmans Welding & Manufacturing Inc.
Phone: 519.765.4230
Email: info@berkelmanswelding.com
Website: www.berkelmanswelding.com

Callicrate Banders
Phone: 785-332-3344
Email: info@nobull.net

Diagnostic Imaging Systems
2325 E. Saint Charles Street
Rapid City, South Dakota
Phone: 605-341-2433
Fax: 605-341-0053
Website: www.vetxray.com

Diamond Farrier Company
361 Haven Hill Road
PO Box 1346
Shelbyville, Kentucky
Phone: 866-844-9622
Fax: 502-633-4168 or 502-633-5863
Website: www.diamondfarrierusa.com

Dr. Bretts Pets – AVTEC Dental
501 Belle Hall Parkway, Ste 201
Mount Pleasure, South Carolina
Phone: 888-688-3855
Email: jen@ivdi.org
Website: drbrettspets.com

iM3 Inc.
122414 NE 95 St
Vancouver, Washington
Phone: 800-664-6348
Website: im3vet.com
Email: info@im3usa.com

Jorgensen Laboratories, Inc.
1450 Van Buren Ave.
Loveland, Colorado
Phone: 970-669-2500 or 800-525-5614
Fax: 970-663-5042
E-mail: info@jorvet.com
Website: www.jorvet.com

Kane Manufacturing
PO Box 413
Perry, Iowa
Phone: 800-247-00038
Website: kanemfg.com
E-mail: info@kanemfg.com

L & H Branding Irons
410 6 St SE
Mandan, North Dakota
Phone: 800-437-8068
E-mail: sales@lhbrandingirons.com
website: https://lhbrandingirons.com/

MacKinnon Products, LLC
1721 Lovall Valley Road
Sonoma, California
Phone: 800-786-6633
Websites: www.Icehorse.net,
www.Hoofwraps.com, www.Sterihoof.com,
www.Tackwrap.com

Miltex, Inc.
1100 Campus Road
Princeton, New Jersey
Phone: 800-645-2873
Fax: 888-980-7742
Website: www.miltex.com

Nasco
901 Janesville Ave.
PO Box 901
Fort Atkinson, Wisconsin
Phone: 920-723-1980 or 800-558-9595
Fax: 800-372-1236
E-mail: custserv@Nascoeducation.com
Website: 855-205-1132
www.nascoeducation.com

Securos Surgical
443 Main Street
PO Box 950
Fiskdale, Massachusetts
Phone: 877-266-3349
eFax: 855-205-1132
Website: www.securos.com

SmartPractice
3400 McDowell Rd
Phoenix, Arizona
Phone: 800-522-0800
Website: smartpractice.com

Stone Manufacturing & Supply Company
1212 Kansas Ave
Kansas City, Missouri
Phone: 816-231-4020
Website: http://www.stonemfg.net/

Sydell, Inc.
46935 SD Highway 50
Burbank, South Dakota
Phone: 800-842-1369
Website: https://sydell.com

Zoetis Animal Health
10 Sylvan Way
Parsippany, New York
Phone: 973-822-7000
Website: zoetis.com

Photo Credits

Photos of the following instruments were provided by
Jorgensen Laboratories, Inc., Loveland, Colorado

Air Bumper Brace
Ambu Bag
Anesthesia and Oxygen Masks
Auspex Avian Positioner
Ayres Non-Rebreathing Circuit
Balfour Retractor
Casey E Collar
Catheter Syringe
Central Venus Catheter—Tear away kit
Corkscrew Trocar
Cornell Detorsion Rod
Cornell Teat Curette
Culture Swab
Dental Chisel
Dental Rasp
Dental Tooth Punch
Doppler Ultrasonic Blood Flow Monitor
Drinkwater Mouth Gags for Cattle
Ear Bulb Syringe
Ecraseur
Electrosurgical Generator
Endotracheal Tube
Enteral Feeding Tubes
Equine Dental Halter
Equine Molar Cutter
Equine Mouth Speculum
Equine Tooth Extractors
Esophagus Stethoscope
Fecal Loop
Fecalyzers
Feeding and Dosing Needles
Fetatome

Fetotomy Knife
Finochietto Rib Spreaders
Fluid Warmer
Foam Neck Brace
Freemartin Probe
Gas Anesthesia Machine
Groove Director
Guardian Touch Vital Signs Monitor
Hauptner Mouse-Ear ID Tags and Applicator
HDE Evolution Power Float Kit—Set 4 Water Cooled
Hemocytometer
Hernia Clamp
Hoof Abscess Knife
Hoof Angle Gauge
Hoof Groover
Hoof Searcher
Inhalation Chamber
Intravenous Drip Sets (Venous Sets)
Intravenous Stand
Jones Towel Forceps
Killian Vaginal Speculum

Krey Obstetrical Hook
Lead Aprons, Gloves, and Thyroid Collars
Lichty Teat Knife or Bistoury
Magnets
Mare Uterine-Flushing Catheter
Mason Meta Splints
Michel Wound Clips
Microcapnograph
Nail Scissors
Nasogastric Feeding Tube
Needle-Sterilizing Rack
Obstetrical Wire Guide
Orthopedic Cast Saw
Pet Piller
Polansky Vaginal Speculum
Purr Muzzle
Radiographic Cassette Holder
Radiographic Hoof Positioner
Rebreathing Bag
Rectal Prolapse Rings
Reimer Emasculator

Roaring Burr
Serra Emasculator
Sheep/Goat Oral Drencher Kit
Simplex Intravenous Bell Sets
Soft E Collar
Stallion Urinary Catheter
Stomach Tube
Tenotome Knife
Thomas-Schroeder Splint
Tourniquet
Tracheostomy Tubes—Small Animal and Equine
Transfer Needle
Trephine (Horsley's)
Vetamatic Dose Syringe
Vulva Suture Pin
White Nail Trimmer
Whites Emasculator
Wire Twister
Wolftooth Elevator

Photos of the following instruments were provided by
Miltex, Inc., York, Pennsylvania
Adson Tissue Forceps
Adson-Brown Tissue Forceps
Alligator Forceps
Allis Tissue Forceps
Babcock Intestinal Forceps
Backhaus Towel Forceps
Beaver Surgical Knife Handles
Castroviejo Needle Holders With Catch
Columbia Curette
Crile Forceps
Dental Elevators
Dressing Forceps
Eye-Dressing Forceps
Ferguson Angiotribe Forceps
Foerster Sponge-Holding Forceps
Gigli Wire Saw and Handles
Half-Curved Tissue Forceps

Halsted Mosquito Forceps
Hartman Mosquito Forceps
Incisor and Root Extracting Forceps
Incisor, Canine, and Premolar Extracting Forceps
Iris Hooks
Iris Scissors
Kelly Forceps
Knowles Bandage Scissors
Lister Bandage Scissors
Mayo Scissors
Metzenbaum Scissors
Molar Extracting Forceps
Operating Scissors
Rochester-Carmalt Forceps
Scalpel Handles
Senn Rake Retractor
Strabismus Scissors
Straight Littauer Stitch Scissors
Weitlaner Retractor
Wire Scissors

Photos of the following instruments were provided by
Nasco, Fort Atkinson, Wisconsin
All-In-One Lamb Castrator, Docker, and Ear Marker
Animal Clippers
Antikick Bar
Ardes Drench Gun—60 mls
Artificial Vagina
Automatic Dose Syringe
Balling Gun
Barnes Dehorner
Bayer Mouth Speculums
Blow Dart
Burdizzo Emasculatome
Calf, Foal, Piglet, Lamb Resuscitators
Calf Snare
Calf Weaners
California Mastitis Test Kit
Cattle Prod
Chain Shank
Clinch Cutter

Cow Boot
Cow Sling
Cribbing Strap/Cradles
Dehorning Saw
Dental Float
Dog Snare or Capture Pole
Drench Pump
Drench-Matic Dose Syringe
Ear Notcher
Elastrator
Equine Mouth Speculum
Ewe Prolapse Retainer
Fabric Show Halter—Cattle
Fabric Show Halter—Sheep
Fetal Extractor (Calf Puller)
Freeze Branding Irons
Frick Speculum
Halter With Lead Rope
Heat-Mount Detector
Hip Lift

Hobbles
Hog Snare
Hoof Blocks
Hoof Knives
Hoof Parer-Pincer
Hoof Pick
Hoof Rasp
Hoof Tester
Hoof Trimmer—Sheep and Goats
Hoof-Trimming Table and Chute
Horn Gouge
Hot-Iron Branding Irons
Insemination Pipettes
Keystone Dehorner (Guillotine)
Labelvage 600-mL Drench Gun
Lambing Instrument
Lariat With Quick-Release Honda
Lead Rope
Long-Handled Hoof Nippers (Squire Hoof Trimmers)
Mare Uterine-Flushing Catheters

Marking Sticks
Milking Tubes
Newberry Castrating Knife
Obstetrical Chains and Handles
Obstetrical Gloves
Oral Calf Drencher
Pig Obstetrical Forceps
Pig Tooth Nipper
Pole Syringe
Restraint Gloves
Rope Halter
Sheep Crook
Sheep-Trimming Shears
Squeeze Chute
Swiss Hoof Knife
Tattoo Outfit—Electric
Tattoo Outfit—Manual—Small Animal and Large Animal
Teat Dilator
Teat Slitter

Teat Tumor Extractor
Thermometer—Digital
Thermometer—Mercury—Small Animal and Large Animal
Trocar and Cannula
Twitch-Chain
Udder-Infusion Cannula
Udder Support
Umbilical Clamp
Umbilical Tape
Whips
White Emasculator
Wire Saw and Handles

Photos of the following instruments was provided by **Allflex/Merk Animal Health, DFW Airport, Texas**
Universal Total Tagger
Visual & FDX EID tag
Tamper Proof Tag

Photo of the following instrument was provided by **Advanced Monitors Corporation, San Diego, California**
  Aural Thermometer (Vet Temp)

Photo of the following instrument was provided by **Arrowquip**, 866-383-7827
  Q Power Hydraulic Chute 104

Photo of the following instrument was provided by **Bella VMS**
  Smart Veterinary Mouth Gag

Photo of the following instrument was provided by **Berkelmans Welding & Manufacturing Inc., 519-765-4230, infor@berkelmanswelding.com**
  Title Table

Photo of the following instrument was provided by Callicrate Banders, info@nobull.net
  Callicrate Bander With Cutter

Photos of the following pieces of equipment were provided by **Diagnostic Imaging Systems, Rapid City, South Dakota**
- Ultra 12030HF Portable Radiography Unit
- Versa View Table
- Chison ECO3 Ultrasound
- DR Wizard ES
- iCR 3600 CR Scanner
- Ultrasound—Wireless and Portable

Photos of the following instruments were provided by **Diamond Farrier Co. Shelbyville, Kentucky**
  Combination Shoe Puller and Spreader
  Crease Nail Puller

Photo of the following instrument was provided by **Dr. Bretts Pets**, drBrettspets.com
  Cacoon Veterinary Dental Handheld X-ray Gun

Photo of the following instrument was provided by
Kane Manufacturing, Perry, Iowa
  Cattle Rattle—Paddle

Photos of the following instruments was provided by
L & H Branding Irons, Mandan, North Dakota
  Universal Branding Iron
  Searing Iron
  Electric Dehorner

Photos of the following instruments were provided by
MacKinnon Products, LLC, Sonoma, California
• Hoof Ice Boot—Horse Therapy Boot

Photo of the following piece of equipment was
provided by Stone Manufacturing & Supply Company
  Henderson Castration Tool

Photo of the following piece of equipment was
provided by Sydell Inc. (www.sydell.com)
• Sheep/Goat Chute—Deluxe Spin Doctor

Photos of the following instruments were provided
by **Securos Veterinary Orthopedics, Fiskdale,
Massachusetts**
  Bone Rasp
  External Fixation Kits
  Intramedullary Pin Chuck
  Intramedullary Pin Cutter
  Intramedullary Pin Setter
  Intramedullary Pins
  Lambert-Lowman Bone Clamp
  Michel Laminectomy Trephine
  Orthopedic Wire

Photo of the following instrument was provided by
SmartPractice, Phoenix, Arizona
  Restraint Air Muzzle II

Photos of the following instruments were provided by
Zoetis, Parsippany, New York
  Vetscan—HM5 Hematology Analyzer
  Vetscan—SA Sediment Analyzer

Vetscan—UA Urine Analyzer
Vetscan—VS2 Chemistry Analyzer
Vetscan—VUE Rapid Test Analyzer
Vetscan—Imagyst

Photos sources from other publications
Close-up photos of the following instruments are from **Nemitz: Surgical Instrumentation: An Interactive Approach, St. Louis, 2009, WB Saunders**.
  Adson Tissue Forceps
  Adson-Brown Tissue Forceps
  Alligator (Wullstein) Forceps
  Castroviejo Needle Holder
  Groove Director
  Halsted Mosquito Forceps
  Iris Scissors
  Lister Bandage Scissors
  Mayo Scissors

Rochester-Péan Forceps
Weitlaner Retractor
Wire Scissors (Angled)

Photo of the following instrument was provided by **Washabau RJ, Day MJ: Canine and Feline Gastroenterology, St. Louis, 2013, Saunders**
Endoscope

Photo of the following instrument was provided by **Sellon DC, Long MT: Equine Infectious Diseases, St. Louis, 2007, Saunders**
  Uterine Cytology Brush

Photo of the following instrument was provided by **Brown M, Brown LC: Lavin's Radiography for Veterinary Technicians, ed 5, St. Louis, 2014, Saunders**
  Hoof-Angle Gauge

Index

Note: Page numbers followed by *f* indicate figures and *t* indicate tables.